Presented to

_____

By

_____

On the Occasion of

_____

Date

_____

D0318630

CONTENTS

IN THE STORM

Precious Lord,
I think I know
a little of what Peter felt
when You called him
to reach beyond himself
and walk on the water,
for I reach too.

I would come to You
unscathed by the storm,
but my faith fails me.
I try to trust
and not let the tumult intimidate,
but worry wrecks my way.

Fear and doubt
assail my dreams,
and it is hard to ignore the raging sea
whipping around me.

Reach for my hand, Father,
lest I sink into the awful waters
and drown in my own fears.

Amen.

Then Peter got down out of the boat, walked on the water and came toward Jesus. But when he saw the wind, he was afraid and, beginning to sink, cried out, "Lord, save me!"

MATTHEW 14:29–30 NIV

One day he got into a boat with his disciples, and he said to them, "Let us go across to the other side of the lake." So they put out, and while they were sailing he fell asleep. A windstorm swept down on the lake, and the boat was filling with water, and they were in danger. They went to him and woke him up, shouting, "Master, Master, we are perishing!" And he woke up and rebuked the wind and the raging waves; they ceased, and there was a calm. He said to them, "Where is your faith?" They were afraid and amazed, and said to one another, "Who then is this, that he commands even the winds and the water, and they obey him?"

LUKE 8:22–25 NRSV

INTRODUCTION

I heard a story once about an art contest where the challenge was to paint a picture depicting peace. Beautiful paintings were submitted of tranquil pastoral scenes, babies serenely asleep in their mother's arms, and many other equally restful sights. The first-place winner, however, depicted a raging storm. A frenzy of the artist's bold brush strokes dominated the canvas. Tree limbs bent under violent wind-driven rain, whitecapped waves pounded hard against the shore, and lightning sliced violently across the black sky. In the lower right-hand corner, amid the chaos, sat a small bird on her nest. Tucked safely under a slightly jutting rock, she remained quiet and calm as she kept her eggs dry and warm.

This said more about peace than all the quiet scenes. That is one of the values of storms, they provide the perfect setting for the nugget of peace or courage or help that prevails. I believe this is because we find God there delivering, guiding, and encouraging us through every storm.

Sometimes the storms are obvious works of

nature. Other times they brew inside us, churning our emotions to the limit. Occasionally the storm is a confrontation between people rather than air masses. We need to remember our God is still there, just as He was with the disciples on that storm-tossed sea so long ago. The question is the same now as it was then. Whatever storm we encounter, it seems to ask, "Where is your faith?"

Stormy Weather

There isn't much that can scare us like a storm. You can't reason your way out of a bad situation when faced with the forces of nature. You can batten down the hatches, you can take cover, or you can attempt to flee; but there is nothing you can do to control bad weather.

That is what makes the story of the disciples caught in the windstorm at sea so amazing. Jesus did the impossible. He calmed the storm just by telling it to stop. His words to His followers give us a clue to the only source stronger than anything we encounter in this natural world.

He didn't tell them they could relax now because He had it all under control. He didn't suggest they should have watched the skies more closely and been better prepared or at least to have awakened Him before it got so bad. At first glance, His response seems strange, even harsh. These were men who knew the sea and what it could do. Surely they had already done everything they could to stay afloat. Yet, He asked them, "Where is your faith?"

His words echo down through the centuries as a strong anchor in present-day storms.

If we face each storm with the idea of looking for our faith somewhere in the chaos and fear, we may not have the waters calmed, but we will have an anchor. And if we develop the habit of finding our faith in every situation, we have something no storm could ever take away.

THE RIDE

An ice storm had kept Jim at work all night for the Pennsylvania Department of Transportation. He drove the large gas truck that kept snowplows supplied with fuel.

Four or five hours of pounding sleet had given the roads a grainy covering that allowed traction. Then a heavy downpour of rain fell on top and turned the road to a smooth sheet of ice. Jim was unaware of the change in texture as he crested a steep hill and headed down just as dawn began to tinge the sky.

At the bottom, the road made a sharp left turn. To miss that turn would mean plunging a vehicle down a two-hundred-foot embankment. He had barely started his descent when he realized he was in trouble. The large truck started to slide sideways, and he shifted to pull out of the skid.

The 2,300-gallon tank was about half full, heavy enough to handle most situations. This time, however, the truck slid out of control.

"Lord, it's all up to You," Jim said aloud as he crossed his arms over his face and laid his head against the steering wheel.

The truck sped over the slippery surface toward the bottom of the hill. Twice, it turned completely around like a spinning top. When it reached the bottom it made the sharp turn and slid to a gentle stop as though guided by unseen hands.

Jim climbed from the truck on shaky legs and looked back up the hill. It surprised him to see no sign of his descent. The rain had turned the sleet into a glassy sheet of ice so hard the heavy truck could not break it.

Was it the angle and pitch of the road that brought a runaway tanker on a treacherous hill to a safe stop? His mother has no question as to how he escaped disaster. Just before daybreak she awoke suddenly from a sound sleep with a strange feeling of concern for her son. "Lord," she prayed, "please be there in the truck with Jim."

FREEZING RAIN

The banshees are coming in crooked
    lines.
I can hear them howling to the north
    in the pines.
Their advance I track
Rattling the bare bones of the trees
Divested of leaves,
In one last attack.

Now they're thrusting their icy spears
Against the windowpane.
I pull up the blankets to cover my ears.
So much for freezing rain.

JEAN ROUNDS

*"I would hurry to find a shelter for myself
from the raging wind and tempest."*
PSALM 55:8 NRSV

TORNADO

When the TV weatherman predicted thunderstorms and a possible tornado watch one morning during a visit with my daughter, Leanne, in Birmingham, Alabama, we canceled plans for a picnic lunch at a park. The rain didn't materialize, however, and by 7:00 P.M. we had forgotten about the forecast.

We became absorbed in a paper Leanne was preparing for a college course she was taking. She needed four copies of the short thesis first thing in the morning and had no way to make them at home. We made a spur of the moment decision to make the twenty-minute drive to the office where she worked three days a week for a company that galvanizes steel. The doors would be locked at nine o'clock, but she figured that should be enough time to get there and type the short paper onto the computer.

Although much of her office area was framed with large glass windows, we didn't notice the darkness or that it had begun to rain. No one knew we were in the deserted building, and the ringing phone startled us.

Leanne's boss was equally surprised when

she answered. He was trying to reach the men working in the production building next door, he quickly explained, to warn them that a tornado was headed eastward. We needed to get out of there as fast as possible, he warned, because we were directly in its path.

When we had arrived about half an hour earlier, the sun had been shining. Now strong wind-driven rain whipped against us as we made our way to the car in the darkness. Leanne turned on the radio as we pulled out of the parking lot. "Everybody take cover. Take cover NOW!" a man's voice barked from the dashboard.

"Do you think we should stop and go into a building somewhere?" I asked as our car crawled through the onslaught of the storm.

"I want to go home," Leanne insisted. I understood. She was a mother, too, and wanted to be with her small son.

The windshield wipers were having a difficult time contending with the torrent of rain. Leanne kept saying, "I can't see. I can't see," and I swiped futilely at the steamy windshield with the palm of my hand.

The worrisome voice on the radio announced that the tornado was traveling at about forty miles per hour. I noted grimly that we weren't doing nearly as well.

My worry button has always had a hair trigger, and risk-taking is for far braver folk than I. The logical left side of my brain considered, in a strangely detached way, that we could die while the right side slid far into disbelief. I don't remember praying. To ask for help would mean admitting the danger, and my mind simply refused to believe there was a tornado bearing down on us. If the clouds had parted and someone said, "Smile, you're on *Candid Camera*," it wouldn't have seemed out of place.

When we reached Leanne's driveway and left the noise of the pounding rain on the metal car, I realized a warning siren was blaring. We grabbed blankets, a radio, and flashlights and gathered in the basement with the rest of the household. After about forty-five minutes the rain subsided, and life resumed its quest for normalcy.

The twister had been a bad one, a Force 5, the worst possible category with winds the experts called "unsurvivable." It wasn't until I bought a newspaper a couple of days later that I realized just how fortunate we had been. It showed the path of the terrible destruction in dark orange.

"Show me where you work," I told Leanne as I handed her the map, "and where is your house?" I stared at the two indentations her fingernail made on the light orange part of the newspaper. The tornado had lifted at a point just short of her workplace and touched down again a little beyond her home. We hadn't outrun it after all. According to the map, it had lifted and hopped right over us.

It is futile to question why we were spared when others weren't. I wish I could say it was an act of faith and a direct answer to our prayers. In truth, however, I was in shock and could not clear my mind of denial that it was actually happening.

I don't know why God chooses to calm some storms and not others. For now, it is enough to know that He can and that He helps us even when we are incapable of asking.

His way is in whirlwind and storm,
and the clouds are the dust of his feet.
NAHUM 1:3 NRSV

Candles in the Wind

For longtime residents of Pell City, a small town about thirty miles east of Birmingham, Alabama, January 10, 1975, is the defining date of their community. They mark time as either before or after the tornado because the town was never the same again.

Though Laura lived in Birmingham with her husband, Jim, she had grown up in Pell City. Her parents still lived there and had operated a store called Red's Men's Wear for many years.

That Friday afternoon Laura sat in a classroom training for a new job. She remained unaware of any weather problems until Jim reached her by phone. He heard on the radio that a tornado had struck her hometown at three o'clock that afternoon.

Unable to reach her parents' store or home by phone, they got in their car and headed east. Although it was only four o'clock, it was dark, and the weather was still rainy and windy.

As their car came closer to Pell City, they began to see signs of damage. Trees were blown down and debris lay scattered on the highway.

Police had barricaded the road into town and were turning people away. Laura was determined, however, to find her parents. Recognizing her as a hometown girl, the authorities reluctantly allowed them to drive past the barricade but warned it was at their own risk.

They managed to reach the high school, where they left the car because the street had become impassable. It was still two miles to her parents' house and farther yet to their Main Street store, where she expected them to be.

They joined with other people on the same mission, looking for loved ones and praying to find them alive. Walking hand in hand, several abreast where possible, they made their way slowly. It was pitch black and still raining lightly. A few people had flashlights, and some light came from occasional lightning flashes and the arcing downed power lines.

The tornado had been an especially bad one, reaching F4 or F5 winds. It was disheartening to make their way down the familiar street. This main street had been lined with century-old oak trees. Most of them had been uprooted or broken, their huge trunks demolishing whatever lay beneath them. Many of the houses were badly damaged. Laura recognized the ruins of former homes of childhood friends and wondered anew how hers had fared.

Here and there the horrible wind seemed to have skipped over a house, causing just minimal damage such as blown-out windows or parts of the roof missing. Some of them, however, were heaps of rubble.

Whenever Laura encountered someone she knew, she asked if they had seen her folks. No one had seen her parents, but finally someone told her, "Your daddy's store is gone." Gone? They would have been working there at three o'clock on a Friday afternoon. Were they gone with the store? she worried.

"Please, God, let us find them." A desperate prayer kept playing over and over in her anxious mind. "Please, God, let them be all right. Please. . ."

When their little group reached the intersection where the street turned down to her parents' home, Laura and Jim turned off alone. It seemed like the longest street Laura had ever walked. Debris was everywhere. Each house they passed had been damaged to some degree.

Laura didn't know what to expect and

hardly dared to let herself think about it as their soggy footsteps took them slowly over and around storm-tossed obstacles in the street. The first thing they noticed was her father's car, crushed like a tin can prepared for recycling from a large tree lying atop it.

They walked around the tree and stood facing the front of the house. It was a one-story cement-block building with no basement. Much of the roof was gone; they could hear it flapping in the wind. In the darkness, however, they could make out the faint glow of two candles flickering in the living room window. Laura had never seen a more welcomed sight in all her life. Someone was there, and they were alive.

Her father met them at the front door. "I knew you'd get here," he said.

Her mother sat in the living room; both parents were in shock. Wind and rain beat inside what was left of their house, but they refused to leave. Laura spent the night on the sofa next to her mother, while Jim and her father sat in chairs. There in the wavering light of the candles, they told their story.

Both of the older people had the flu, and in an almost unheard-of act, they left the store early and came home. That decision alone probably saved their lives. They later found only three walls still standing where the store had been. An eight hundred-pound air conditioner had been carried many miles, and new shirts, still in their packages with the store's tags on them, were found as far as sixty miles away.

They had no warning of the tornado. If they had an alarm system for the town back then, it wasn't working. It had grown dark and started raining and thundering, they remembered. The wind blew hard, so hard, in fact, that it blew the back door open. Laura's mother automatically hurried to close it.

Fortunately, Laura's father responded differently. He could only explain that something told him to get her out of there. He ran after his wife, grabbed her arm, and pulled her quickly into the bathroom. There, he pushed her down to the floor and shielded her body with his own. It was over quickly.

In its wake, the storm left its savage mark. The back half of the house was completely destroyed. An enclosed porch, two bedrooms, and a breakfast area, along with all the furniture and a washing machine, had been battered by the terrible wind. The cement blocks were crumbled.

They shuddered to think of the what-ifs. What if they hadn't been sick and come home? Would they have vanished with the store? What if Laura's mother had continued on her way to close the back door? They had no doubt she would have been sucked into that swirling mass.

In spite of the extreme damage to their properties, they had a lot to be grateful for. To this day, Laura carries an image of hope in her mind of two tiny candles flickering in the wind.

Storm at Night

My room's alight from the lightning flash.
I wait for the following sound.
The house trembles with the thunder's crash,
And the rain comes tumbling down.

Nature's determined to vent her wrath,
But here inside it's dry and warm.
I lie awake listening to this rainy bath,
My room an oasis in the storm.

"Though the rain comes in torrents, and the floods rise and the storm winds beat against his house, it won't collapse. . . ."

Matthew 7:25 TLB

The Flood

Hurricane Agnes brought an incredible amount of rain to the northeastern part of Pennsylvania, where my parents and two younger brothers lived in June of 1972. Although they knew it was coming, as weathermen carefully charted the hurricane's path, no one was prepared for the extent of the flooding.

Mom listened to the radio that morning after my stepfather left for work around seven o'clock. The weather report warning of heavy rain and flooding prompted her to check the situation for herself. She put on her coat and walked about a quarter of a mile to the nearest creek.

The normally trickling stream had grown fairly high with the rapid rush of muddy floodwaters, but it was still contained within its banks. A farmer's field and a several-foot-high embankment that supported the highway stood between the creek and Mom's yard. Although high, the flooding didn't seem to pose much of a threat at that point. The river was another mile away from the stream.

As she made the short walk back home, however, she was shocked at the intensity of the rain. She had never seen it pour so hard. It felt as though a giant spigot had been turned on in the sky.

Kevin, the younger of my two teenaged brothers, was still asleep when she returned to the house. She felt nervous enough to awaken him and suggest they drive his Bronco to check out the river. Elwyn, the nineteen year old, was at work. Mom's fears were confirmed when she saw the rapidly rising waters, and the rain just kept on falling in torrents.

My stepfather returned around noontime and, with the help of a friend, pulled the pump from the well. By 4:00 P.M. the garden, with onions and peas almost ready to pick, was covered, and the roily water inched across the lawn toward the house.

Kevin had gone to his part-time job at a gas station on the other side of the river, and by late afternoon, he was needed at home to help move things to higher ground. The phone lines were down, so my mother decided to go get him with her car.

The river had reached fearsome proportions and driving across the bridge frightened her. When she reached the gas station, however, she discovered he had already left for home.

Mom returned home the way she had come, crossing the bridge again with her heart in her mouth. Kevin, however, chose a different way and crossed a bridge further up the river. It was an old structure, and the angry water slammed hard against the abutment while it splashed close to the underside of the floor.

C. S. Lewis once wrote: "If we could see all our guardian angels around us, we'd get claustrophobic." I always felt Kevin needed all the guardian angels heaven could muster because he was a risk-taker. That day on the bridge was one of those times. He pushed the Bronco's gas pedal to the floor and tore over that stressed structure as fast as he could. He was the last one to cross. Shortly afterward, the remnants of a floating building slammed the bridge broadside, and it collapsed into the raging floodwaters.

Neighbors who lived further up the hill came without being asked and pitched in to help move furniture and appliances to higher ground. It was a race against time as everyone hurried to snatch what they could from the jaws of the hungry river.

The washer, dryer, and freezer were taken to a neighbor's barn, while everything in lower cupboards was placed on the countertops. Photographs and sentimental knickknacks were moved upstairs.

As they vacated the house they heard meowing and remembered the three cats who stayed in one of the outbuildings. Three feet of water had lifted the small shed from its concrete base, and it was beginning to float. Elwyn rowed a small boat, while Kevin waded inside. Three terrified cats had climbed to the top of a pile of hay bales. When they saw their rescuer, they frantically climbed Kevin's body like a tree trunk and clung there as he waded outside to the rowboat.

Mom had moved her car to the top of the hill behind the house. The four of them huddled there throughout the night—wet, hungry, and heartsick. Kevin, soaked from rescuing the cats, was wrapped up in a blanket that happened to be in the car. Mom, in her panic, had grabbed two quarts of home-canned tomatoes and totally forgotten a chicken roasting in the wall oven.

They watched the water slowly begin to swallow their home, and when darkness finally closed in, it was halfway up the first story. The local radio station stayed on the air all night long broadcasting information on the rising waters and passing on the pleas of people desperately trying to locate missing relatives. Their home might be invaded by a smelly, muddy mess, but at least they were together.

Daylight showed the water about halfway up the house. The high-water mark would eventually prove to be about one inch from the first-floor ceiling. They stayed with neighbors for a couple of days until they could go back and begin the major job of drying out and cleaning.

One moment of panic came the second day into the flood. Word came that a dam several miles to the north was near the breaking point. If they wanted to save anything more, they were warned, they had better do it quickly.

Mom, Kevin, and a neighbor took the rowboat and made their way to the house, where they managed to dock at the eaves on the side porch. They crawled into the house through an upstairs bedroom window. A glance down the stairway was a disheartening sight. Articles that had, just yesterday, been a normal part of their household surroundings now floated over the stairs. Plastic bowls, a wooden spoon, and the dining room table had become debris.

What to save? What to leave behind? They hurriedly grabbed pictures, jewelry, and any other item they could safely carry in the small boat. Fortunately the dam held and the tough choices proved unnecessary.

Cleanup was a major undertaking. The muddy water left silt on everything it touched. After the fire company pumped the basement, it proved easier to eventually concrete over the sediment than to remove it. The firemen also lent them a machine called a salamander that ran for days on end, filling the downstairs rooms with warm arid air to help them dry.

The most tedious work was the nitty-gritty cleaning. Kitchen cupboards were full of food that had spent two days soaking in filthy water. Flour had become a sticky paste, macaroni had turned to gunk, and oatmeal was slime. Their home had turned into a seed-bed for disease, and everyone had to have shots to prevent typhoid and cholera.

Times such as these sharpen one's awareness of blessings, and over and over you could hear someone say, "It could have been worse." Crisis brings out the best in people, and the bigger the storm, the bigger the response. Neighbors my folks had never met came and took curtains, draperies, and clothing home to wash. Strangers from out of the area arrived and rolled up their sleeves to help those who had been victims. They scrubbed and hosed and carried trash. They brought food, water, cleaning supplies, and hugs.

Someone gave Mom a snapshot that had been taken at the time of the flood. It was a picture of dark clouds wind-driven in such a way that it looked like Jesus coming down out of them. It gave a visual aid to what they had already found. It was a terrible storm, but they never for an instant had to endure it alone.

The LORD sits enthroned over the flood;
the LORD is enthroned as King forever.
The LORD gives strength to his people;
the LORD blesses his people with peace.
PSALM 29:10–11 NIV

God will put his angels in charge of you
to protect you wherever you go.

PSALM 91:11
GOOD NEWS BIBLE

ANGELS OF THE SNOW

JoAnne knew she probably shouldn't be out in the snowstorm. With her bad back and knee problems, she had trouble enough on good firm ground. It would take only a few minutes to pull up near the small-town library, however, and navigate the short walkway to the drop box. Those books really should go back, she reasoned with herself.

She made it to the drop box, but on the way back, her feet slipped out from under her, and she plunged into a pile of deep snow. Her efforts to pull herself out made her feel like she was in quicksand. She just seemed to sink deeper.

Her cries for help went unheard. Visibility was bad with the windblown heavy flakes, and the parts of her coat and hat that weren't buried in the snowbank were covering so quickly they began to blend in with the storm. Her mind started to panic with thoughts of dying right there on Main Street.

Then, like a vision from heaven, a woman's face hovered over her and was immediately joined by a man. They were going by in their car, the woman told JoAnne, and caught a glimpse of her lying in the snow.

They pulled JoAnne to her feet and walked her to her car. She was so upset by then that she forgot to even ask them their names. She still refers to them as her guardian angels—her angels in the snow.

SNOWFLAKE

Look!
On the sleeve of my coat,
the tiniest miracle,
one snowflake,
a miniature cathedral window.

CORINNE CRONLUND

Snowstorms can be welcomed if you like the opportunity for play they offer or a marvel of beauty when viewed from inside a cozy home.

Travel on snow-covered roads, however, is a different story, especially when that storm grows to blizzard proportions. My best friend, Helen, wrote the following account in her journal back in 1982 and has graciously agreed to let me share it.

THE BLIZZARD

My husband, Carlton, and I had just spent the last week in February on vacation in Florida and reluctantly packed our car to head home to Pennsylvania. It was raining, but the forecast kept telling us it was going to turn to freezing rain and snow. We were in the southern states; certainly we could handle a little snow. After all, look where we lived. We figured we were used to it.

When we stopped for dinner, we tried to call ahead for reservations for the night, but all the motels were full. Other diners who were headed south told us of freezing rain ahead of us, so we got a room and spent the night right where we were.

Sunday morning we scraped ice off the windshield and started out again. The interstate was slippery, but by driving accordingly we made pretty good time. Then it began to snow.

When we stopped for lunch, we decided we had better not try to go as far as Richmond that night, as we had planned, and made reservations at a closer place instead. The clerk promised to hold our room until 6:00 P.M. We thought we could easily be there by four o'clock.

Our waitress told us the forecast had changed, and they were now predicting six to eight inches of snow. We filled the car with gas and started out again. It never occurred to us that we should stay right where we were even though great big flakes were coming down hard. With good snow tires on a main highway, we didn't think we should have any problem. We had driven in worse situations back home and took it all in stride.

It didn't take us long, however, to realize we were headed for trouble. We kept telling each other it would probably stop any minute, but the snow came down harder and the wind started to blow. We soon came upon cars and tractor-trailers here and there that had slid over into the median. When we passed a big eighteen-wheeler completely overturned, I really began to worry.

I studied the map for a place to stop but found we were in a very desolate area. It was getting very difficult for Carlton to drive. Ice forming on the windshield and thick snow made it difficult for him to see the road. Even so, there was still the occasional crazy driver who sped past us, creating a whirlwind of snow behind him.

It was risky to keep going, but it was even more dangerous to stop. If we pulled off to the side of the road, there was too much risk of being hit. Each exit ramp we came upon was so full of snow we couldn't use it. There was nowhere to go, even if we had been able to get off. According to my map, what few towns there were, were at least twenty miles away.

We knew we would never make it to our reserved room. All we wanted at that point was to get off the highway and find a place to stay. By then, there was only one lane of traffic and nearly zero visibility.

We came upon two cars stuck in the right lane with a man trying to slow traffic. We managed to edge by him, as did the car behind us. I could see in my rearview mirror that the third car went over onto the median. Then I watched in horror as a tractor-trailer came up quickly in the left lane with another one slightly behind him in the right. They couldn't stop, and I saw the man leap over the bank. A sudden gust of wind created a whiteout, and I could no longer see any of them.

"Oh, God," I prayed desperately, "please keep everyone safe and help us get off this highway."

I tried to study the map, watch for stalled vehicles, and pray as hard as I could all at the same time. Suddenly I saw a sign that said there was a Howard Johnson Motel eight miles up the road. There was no Gold Rock, North Carolina, listed on my map, but sure enough, we found the exit. It appeared just about everybody else on that highway had the same idea, and traffic was backed up on the ramp from cars stuck in the unplowed snow.

Carlton pulled over as far as he could and decided to scrape the windshield. He took the key out of the ignition to open the trunk to get his hat and gloves, and when he tried to restart the car, the battery was dead.

He told me to stay with the car while he went to get help. A man in a pickup truck gave him a lift. I kept on praying. We weren't safe, parked where we were, and I didn't even have a flashlight. I remembered the accident I had seen earlier and was afraid I would be hit any minute.

A truck came up the ramp the wrong way and stopped right in front of me. There were four young fellows in it, and they asked me what was wrong. I told them the car was dead. One of them said he was sorry, but he didn't have any jumper cables. Well, I did, I told him, and I didn't waste any time getting them out of my trunk.

They soon had my car running, but I knew I could never drive it off the ramp. I couldn't even see the road. One of the young men drove it for me. They were having a great time and making a lot of money helping stranded travelers like me.

I was grateful to be off the highway, but there I sat at the end of the exit ramp. "Oh, God," I prayed, "what do I do now? I don't know where Carlton is. The storm is worse than ever and there are cars stuck everywhere I look."

I knew I had to move the car, so I jumped into the driver's seat. When I looked up, Carlton was running toward me. I said a quick prayer of thanks for one more solved problem.

We pulled into the motel's parking lot, and there were cars everywhere. We knew there would be no vacant rooms, but what about a parking place? I told Carlton there looked to be one near the door and wondered why no one had taken it. As we drew closer we found the wind had made a huge drift across the space. Carlton pulled in anyway and ran right through it. We were safe. It was 6:00 P.M.

We stayed with about 250 other stranded travelers, sleeping in a banquet room with about 50 of them. We were lucky enough to get a mattress pad, a sheet, and two pillows.

The floor was hard. "But, oh, God," I prayed, "I can put up with that. We're warm and safe with food and shelter. Please, Father, be with all those other people who are caught out in this terrible storm."

The morning newspaper said thirty-six people died in North Carolina in that blizzard. I felt deeply grateful to God that, with His graciousness, our failure to heed the warning signs hadn't made it thirty-eight.

God moves in a mysterious way
His wonders to perform;
He plants his footsteps in the sea
And rides upon the storm.

WILLIAM COWPER

*Now give orders for your livestock and
everything else you have in the open to
be put under shelter. Hail will fall. . . .*

EXODUS 9:19
GOOD NEWS BIBLE

THE HAILSTORM

Hail is mentioned several times in the Bible, usually in fearsome passages of the prophets predicting doom and destruction. After experiencing only one of these frightening storms, I can see why it is a force to be feared.

I was home alone that late spring day. It was a Saturday afternoon, and my three children had gone their separate ways with friends or to part-time jobs. My son, Mark, had taken several of his friends for a drive in our station wagon. I took advantage of the quiet house to sit peacefully in my bedroom and catch up on some reading.

Absorbed in my book, I was unaware of any weather changes outside until I heard the first heavy raindrops begin to plop on the patio roof beneath my window. Spring showers, the kind that bring the proverbial May flowers, are a welcomed sound, but this one quickly turned nasty.

Hail began to mix with the raindrops and made sharp pinging sounds as it bounced off the roof. The pinging soon turned more ominous. The size of the hailstones became increasingly large and the noise proportionately louder. Mark surprised me when he came rushing into my room because I hadn't heard him come home. He was wet and rubbing sore spots where he had been hit with the icy pellets when he ran from the garage to the house. His friends were still inside the car, he explained, but he hadn't wanted me to be alone.

I was soon glad he had chosen to be so thoughtful. The noise grew alarming. We stared at each other in disbelief as the sound amplified until it reminded me of a train driving across the rooftop. I had heard of hail sometimes described as golf-ball size but had never seen it firsthand. The lawn turned white as it became covered with millions of these dangerous balls of ice.

It lasted only a few minutes, but the damage it wreaked was astonishing. I felt glad I hadn't planted my garden yet because it would have been destroyed. As it was, the rhubarb leaves and stalks lay pummeled into the ground. The new leaves on the maple tree covered the yard as though it were autumn. We raked the shredded leaves and twigs for days.

Fortunately, the insurance company paid to repair the few holes poked in the roof, and my car had been spared by Mark getting it into the garage before the worst of the storm hit. A lot of other people weren't nearly as lucky.

The kids gathered some of the biggest pieces of ice and put them in the freezer for proof of their size and future bragging rights.

It's easy to read a piece of Scripture until it feels flat. It will be a long time, however, before I read about hailstones and not be sufficiently impressed.

Praise the Lord from the earth,
sea monsters and all ocean depths;
lightning and hail, snow and clouds,
strong winds that obey his command.

PSALM 148:7–8
GOOD NEWS BIBLE

Heavenly Creator, how awesome are Your ways.
I tremble in Your presence and at Your mighty
works of nature. You speak with the voice
of thunder and blow a blizzard's breath
across the land. You call the stars by name.
I am humbled and fearful of Your majesty.
And yet, You number the hairs on my head
and speak in a still, small voice to my heart.
I am overwhelmed that You consider me at all.
I am as insignificant as a drop of water in the
ocean of Your creation, but still You bother
with my puny life and call me Your child.
There are no words great enough to capture
what that means to me. I have to settle
for thank You and trust You to understand.
Amen.

Since I started writing this book, I've become acutely aware of storms. Today nature put on a glorious performance, and I was struck anew by the artistry of such events.

At first I refused to be drawn by curiosity to watch because I was busy at my computer. A slight flicker of the lights, however, and I shut down my electronic gadgets to observe the master electrician in action. My front door has a full-length glass storm door, so I sat down on the carpeted entranceway and watched the show.

Distant thunder heralded the event, growing louder as the sky turned darker. Lightning flicked like serpents' tongues from the clouds. It made me remember how, as children, we used to calculate the progress of a storm by determining the time between lightning flash and thunder. We used the kid-approved scientific method of one-Mississippi, two-Mississippi, three-Mississippi.

Raindrops began to fall in a straight-down fashion until the storm worked to a fevered pitch of wind. Gusts swept sheets of rain across my front yard. Then, big hams that storms can be, came the hail. The icy marble-sized balls quickly polka-dotted the lawn as they fell and bounced, resembling Mexican jumping beans.

Thunder crashed like large artillery and vibrated somewhere inside my chest cavity. No Mississippi in that one! It's impossible to remain unaffected by a thunderstorm.

The hail marked the crescendo of this magnificent symphony, and the rain soon settled into a steady drizzle. Alabama, where I live, is in the throes of a drought, so the longer the drizzle the better, at this point. A drizzle, however, is not star material, so I got to my feet to go back to work. I could still hear thunder rolling off into the distance, announcing this Sunday afternoon matinee for some other neighborhood.

Thank You, God, for this awesome reminder of just how great You are. Bravo!

STORMY WEATHER PRAYER

Creator God, Your world is an awesome place,
especially when nature unleashes its power.
It is at times like these that we remember
just how fragile our existence is on this planet

where we so smugly claim dominion.
It takes just one brush with a furious storm
to send us scurrying in our minds for refuge
with the only greater power we know, Lord.
Thank You for accepting us as little children
and holding us firm to ride out the storm.
                                        Amen.

In my distress I cry to the Lord, that he
may answer me. . . .

PSALM 120:1 NRSV

Inner Storms

Inner storms can be as dangerous and destructive as the forces of nature. Anger, grief, worry, anxiety, doubt, depression, fear, guilt, stress. . . these internal disturbances rock the foundation of our being and dictate our behavior. Instead of raindrops, they bring tears; rather than thunder, they produce harsh words and actions. Like a blizzard, they chill the heart; and with the force of a whirlwind, they can tear us apart.

Inner storms are not always obvious. At times they resemble the water bird that sails serenely across the pond but paddles like crazy beneath the surface. A sunny smile has been known to mask a deluge inside.

The Bible addresses these storms. Lamentations 3:22 (NIV) assures us, "Because of the LORD's great love we are not consumed, for his compassions never fail." From Psalm 73:26 (NRSV) come the comfortable words, "My flesh and my heart may fail, but God is the strength of my heart and my portion forever."

Some of the most reassuring words against the storms of life come from Jesus in Matthew 11:28–29 (NIV), "Come to me, all you who are weary and burdened, and I will give you rest. Take my yoke upon you and learn from me, for I am gentle and humble in heart, and you will find rest for your souls."

Inner storms make us question our own worth and our relationship with our creator and sustainer. From deep within our souls we ask ourselves, "Where is my faith?"

Lay aside every weight and the sin that clings so closely, and let us run with perseverance the race that is set before us. . . .
HEBREWS 12:1 NRSV

LETTING GO OF THE GARBAGE

I slid a paring knife under the thin plastic label as I prepared a soda bottle for recycling. Most peeled off, except for one small strip, which I removed with my thumb and forefinger.

When I held it over the waste can and opened my fingers, static electricity made it cling to the side of my thumb. I pulled it off with the other hand only to have it stick to that one. Back and forth I pulled it from hand to hand. I simply could not get rid of this small piece of garbage.

That little strip of plastic has a lot in common with the garbage in my life. Life's storms bring worry, guilt, and fear that threaten my faith in myself and, even worse, my faith that God will see me through. My thoughts run in circles, and my stomach churns as I struggle with feelings that immobilize me, similar to the inactive electrons that make up static electricity. I cling to them, and the static keeps me from running the best race I can.

I hit one of those it-never-rains-but-what-it-pours points in my life recently, and the stress from multiple problems inflicted me with odd bouts of nausea. I felt as though my prayers for resolution had been put on hold at some heavenly switchboard. Surely God wasn't listening, or worse yet, didn't care about my troubles or me.

At my lowest point, an unexpected E-mail note arrived from a faraway friend who had no idea of anything that was transpiring in my little storm-drenched world. "He calmed the raging sea," she wrote, "and can calm your little old stomach"—I hadn't told anyone about my upset stomach—"and put more thoughts into your mind than you could ever imagine. He is only a whisper away." She ended, "Isn't that the wonder of it all?"

I don't know why she wrote what she did, but it came at just the right time and calmed my tempest in a teapot that felt like the raging sea to me. It was just what I needed to be told at that moment.

Just as I salvaged the soda bottle and kept it from becoming landfill, God saves our lives from becoming buried in garbage too. For the soda bottle, it's called recycling; Christians call it salvation. Salvation is a very nice noun, but we use it so much, the cutting edge has worn smooth. It slides right over us sometimes like other popular words do, words like "love," or "how are you," or "have a nice day."

As a writer, I've grown to value verbs. They're tough little guys that get the job done and give teeth to a manuscript. The verb of salvation is salvage. It is a word of Old French origin, and the dictionary gives one meaning as "the saving of any goods from destruction or waste." Salvage is also what they call it when a sunken ship or its cargo is rescued from the depths.

Part of the verse from Psalm 31:12 (Good

News Bible) reads, "I am like something thrown away." Inner storms can make us feel that way sometimes. They undermine our self-confidence and self-worth and make us feel ready for the garbage heap. Fortunately for us, we belong to a God who salvages lives when we are ready to throw them away.

THE STREETLIGHT

The streetlight in front of our house had burned out, and I didn't know how to go about getting the bulb replaced. Was it a problem to take to the town council, or did one report it to the electric company? I simply knew I didn't have time to bother with it.

Besides, the only time I really missed it was the one night a week I worked late at a doctor's office. On those nights I fumbled with my door key in the near darkness and vowed halfheartedly to check into the matter tomorrow. Of course, I never did.

Like everyone else, I juggled a too-full schedule. My life reminded me of the circus performer who keeps several plates spinning on sticks, racing to each one to set it spinning again before it can tumble and shatter. Job. Family. House. Church. I divided my time and energy until sometimes all my "plates" wobbled badly. I felt as burned-out as that streetlight.

Once a week for over a month I kept telling myself I needed to do something about that absent light that made such a difference on a dark night at the end of our little dead-end street. It was inevitable I would put it off too long.

I had a meeting that ran late, and my husband was out of town. I was only about fifteen miles from home, but I felt like I had stumbled into the opening of a bad novel that began, "It was a dark and stormy night. . . ."

Hard rain and wind blew the October leaves onto the wet road and made visibility poor. For several miles the roadway bordered a desolate area by a swamp. I didn't like the drive on a good day. That night it gave me the creeps. Then the car started making a strange sound, and I had visions of getting stranded. By the time I reached the edge of my hometown, I had worked myself into a good case of the jitters.

Even though I made it home safely, I realized I had to go from the garage to the house and unlock the front door in rain and darkness. How I wished I had called someone about that miserable streetlight.

When I pulled down our short street, however, I smiled. "They fixed the light," I said aloud to the empty car, "and on a Saturday."

I didn't think any more about it after being grateful for the well-lit walkway and front porch. A few days later I picked some parsley from my garden and took it to my next-door neighbors, an older couple. We had visited for awhile at their door when the husband asked, "How do we get that streetlight fixed?"

"I thought it was fixed," I responded.

"Well, it did come on for just one night," he answered, "but that was all."

One night. The night I needed it most. Why did I worry so much about my spinning plates? I wondered as I walked back to my house. I was in the care of the One who spins the universe. Who could ask for anything more?

WORRY

Flashes of panic
skitter across my mind
like heat lightning
teasing the horizon.

Tossed in a tempest
of thought,
I pray to the One who calms the sea
to still the storm in me.

ANGER

Hot words.
Cold voice.
Cool stare.
Warm tears.

WHO DO YOU SAY THAT I AM?

I don't know what to call You.
Father?
Lord?
God?
Jehovah?

I only know that my heart
reaches for Your heart.
Shaky.
Unsure.
Groping.

I don't know Your name,
only that I reach.

Into each life some rain must fall,
Some days must be dark and dreary.
HENRY WADSWORTH LONGFELLOW

*"He will wipe away all tears from their
eyes. There will be no more death, no
more grief or crying or pain. The old
things have disappeared." Then the one
who sits on the throne said, "And now I
make all things new!"*
REVELATION 21:4–5
GOOD NEWS BIBLE

Making Things New

The sky was leaden, and it matched my mood as I stood and stared out the window. Autumn winds had stripped the maple limbs bare and tossed her seed wings to the wind. The empty limbs matched the dead brown grass.

Birds darted to the feeder for seeds in an effort to beat the gathering storm. I watched the activity before me, but my thoughts were really with Sandy and how like the desolate winter landscape her life had become.

She was part of a patchwork of adolescent memories—maypole dances, shorthand classes, high school graduation. We had been friends since we were twelve, and now she had leukemia. Her family scurried like these birds to squeeze more from her final weeks before dark clouds rolled in forever.

Crystal flakes began to fall quickly as I brooded at the window, and within minutes everything turned white. Hemlock boughs donned snow-lace coats, and the lawn turned pristine. Every stark limb of the maple tree became edged in a perfect white outline. Even the weathered old bird feeder sparkled. The pure beauty brought a lump to my throat as it occurred to me that I had to let Sandy go and trust her to the One who not only made all things new, but made them incredibly beautiful.

OUTPOURING

No crocodile tears, these.
They are pouring from the reservoir of
    my being
Through the broken dam of my heart.

Somehow, I must shore up the broken part
Until I can find the energy to start
    rebuilding.
The question is how, where to start?

JEAN ROUNDS

Storms are a natural part of nature, just as conflict and difficulty are a natural part of living. Sometimes we take life too seriously and it takes something as elemental as a storm to give us wisdom.

In his sermon today, our pastor told about a young man who yearned to know the meaning of life. He struggled with this monumental question alone for a while without success. Finally he asked his rabbi if he would teach him this truth. After careful thought, the rabbi agreed.

"The next time it rains, I want you to go out and stand in the downpour," the old man told him. The next time the skies opened up and sent rain, the obedient student did as he had been instructed and stood in the torrent.

"What did you learn?" the wise teacher asked.

"All I learned was that I got wet," the disappointed young man replied.

"That is enough for the first lesson," the rabbi said and nodded.

Thank You, Lord, for the storms that put our lives in perspective and shower us with a dose of reality.

RAIN SONG

It's raining out tonight,
A warm, gentle friendly rain,
Kissing each stalk of hay
A hundred times.

It plays comforting rhymes
Upon tin roofs
And milk can lids.
I hope it lingers on,
Perhaps 'til dawn,
For tonight,
I need a friend to cry with.

LE STANTON

*I waited patiently for God to help me;
then he listened and heard my cry. He
lifted me out of the pit of despair, out
from the bog and the mire, and set my
feet on a hard, firm path and steadied
me as I walked along. He has given me a
new song to sing, of praises to our God.*

PSALM 40:1–3 TLB

A PSALM FOR DEPRESSION

It has been said that depression is anger turned inward. When that particular malady struck me, God placed in my life a wise doctor to help me weather the angry storm brewing inside me by writing my way through it.

She called it homework. This gentle woman said I had lost the ability to feel happiness when I came to her for help. "Write down what you're thinking," she directed, "and bring it to me each week."

The first time I met with her she asked me to explain why I had come, and I answered, "When I was a little girl and scowled or pouted, my grandmother would ask, 'What if your face froze that way?' Well, I have become very unhappy, and I feel like I've frozen that way, for I can't feel anything else." Like the writer of Psalm 40, my life had sunk into "the bog and the mire."

She agreed I had lost the ability to feel happiness but felt sure she could help me overcome this sickness of sadness. When she learned I used to write before circumstances beyond my control sent my life tumbling downward into that "pit of despair," she sent me back to the typewriter.

For eighteen months I wrote my way to emotional health. My tears sometimes fell onto the keys as I imparted the desolation and pain. At other times anger hammered across the paper when I wrestled with the hopeless, helpless, and worthless feelings of the illness.

From the vantage point of several years' of hindsight, now I realize God was always there. At the time, however, He had grown silent, and my faith seemed to have failed me. "Is there a God?" I wrote in my homework one day. "And does He believe in me?"

Another time I typed, "I try so hard to get well. People keep asking me about my writing. 'Are you still writing? Have you written any more poetry? When are you going to write something?' I hate it! I'm not writing. I can't write anymore. That's all in the past. It's gone, gone, GONE! If one more person mentions my talent, I may explode. I don't have any talent. I can barely think coherently."

This wise doctor never refuted my typed tirades. She always just smiled as she eagerly reached out her hand for my weekly pile of pages and urged me to do more.

Gradually tiny triumphs, so small to barely be noticed, crept into my journal (for that is what it was, a journal of a journey through the blackness). "I bought a few seeds," I told my typewriter one day. "I'll plant a small garden and not neglect it like last year. I used to be a pretty good gardener. My shelf of writer's books sits untouched for a long time now. I don't know if my creative ability is dormant or dead. Is it one of the shattered things that can be put back together again? I feel like I'm refurnishing a room, only it's inside me. If this room can't be filled with good pieces, then it is better to leave it empty. Maybe I can draw some satisfaction from my handful of seeds and try to forget I once cultivated hopes and dreams instead."

Slowly, God lifted me to set my feet on firm ground. "I feel a pinprick of hope stirring," one of the later pages read. "It's a tiny glimmer of light like a distant star trying to pierce a cloudy night. I can base it on nothing concrete. It's just a feeling, and it is good. But then, that's the stuff hope grows on. Absolutes don't need hope."

Before my illness I lacked the self-confidence to call myself a writer, even though I had been published in magazines. I would say, "I write," and leave it at that. Then the depression swallowed me, and I thought I would never write again. I realize now that I never actually stopped.

Although I felt God had turned away from me, He was catching my tears and lavishing mercy. He held me in His hand like a quill pen dipped in the ink of human misery. With His steadfast love and faithfulness holding me safe, I wrote my way to wellness and beyond. That is the new song He gave me to sing, or, in my case, the new story He gave me to write. Now, when anyone asks, "Are you a writer?" I'm not afraid to tell them yes.

DOUBT

Believe.
The word thunders down
through the centuries.

Believe
and possess the key
that opens impossibilities.
I hold up my flimsy faith,
tattered with questions
and uncertainty.

I whisper prayers
and hope
someone listens.

I pursue goodness
and pray
that it matters.

I struggle with a slippery will
and lose
and wonder if God is watching.

Believe.
God is everywhere.
He shouldn't be hard to find.

Yet,
through the dark chambers of my soul,
walk fear and confusion.
With my tiny candle
of belief,
I tread there too.

A man who carries a cat by the tail
learns something he can learn
in no other way.

MARK TWAIN

*For my thoughts are not your thoughts,
nor are your ways my ways, says the
Lord. For as the heavens are higher than
the earth, so are my ways higher than
your ways and my thoughts than your
thoughts.*

ISAIAH 55:8–9 NRSV

MARGRATEN

Storm clouds looming on the horizon quickened our pace. The most pressing thought on my mind as we pulled into the parking lot at Margraten was to hurry through this little military cemetery in the Netherlands before the rain caught up with us and ruined my hairdo.

My son, Mark, was finishing a ten-month stay as an exchange student in Aachen, Germany; my mother and I flew over to spend the last two weeks with him. We had a full itinerary as we tried to cram as much as possible into this trip of a lifetime.

Ever since Mark and his English friend, Jane, met us at the Frankfurt airport with a long-stemmed rose for each of us, we had been in a holiday spirit. Everything became an adventure while we toured ancient Roman ruins and museums, explored quaint little shops for unique souvenirs, and sampled new foods at sidewalk cafes. We rode one of Germany's high-speed trains, hiked through villages with storybook settings, and snapped pictures of castles and vineyards as we cruised the Rhine River.

We found humor in every new experience, with three generations teasing each other's attempts at absorbing a different culture. They laughed at me when we saw a windmill in the distance. Who could resist a windmill in Holland? I insisted we take a closer look. After a few wrong turns, we finally located the interesting structure and were delighted to find it was open to the public. We happily paid the admission fee only to discover it housed an exhibit of live spiders, my greatest phobia. I couldn't even look at their picture in the encyclopedia without feeling creepy. My stay inside the windmill was extremely brief, but it was enough to provide my family with years of laughter.

We tried to accommodate everyone's wishes. Mine had been chasing windmills; Mom's was Margraten, a small plot of land tucked into the gently rolling hills near the

German border. It was given to the United States by the people of the Netherlands as a place to bury the men and women who died there in WWII.

Our German host tried to dissuade us. "Why would anyone want to visit a graveyard when there were so many other things to do?" he asked in wonder. My mother held firm. She remembered the war and some of the young men who never came home again.

We could see it meant a lot to her, and it wouldn't take long to stop by on our way to a city in the Netherlands that Mark wanted us to see. A quick stop there to make Mom happy and we could spend the rest of the day shopping and strolling the streets of an intriguing foreign city.

That was my frame of mind as Mark, Jane, Mom, and I walked quickly from the parking lot toward the cemetery entrance. Hurry. Do this for Mom. Hurry. It's going to rain. Hurry. I don't want to get wet. Hurry. Hurry. Hurry!

Wide white marble steps brought us first to a beautiful little square with a reflection pool in the center and white walls flanking both sides. It was a place that suggested peace and tranquility, but the storm was coming, and we hurried toward another set of steps at the opposite end.

I was totally unprepared for the emotion that seized me the moment I stepped across the threshold of those few steps and saw eight thousand white crosses all in perfect rows. The silence was complete, and I felt as though time had come to an abrupt halt. "Oh, God, no!" a voice cried deep inside me, and I blinked hard to fight back the tears.

We had seen remnants of the Siegfried line (the sawtooth-shaped chunks of concrete meant as barriers to stop tanks from crossing from France into Germany during the war), and in the woods near our bed-and-breakfast was a large, bowl-shaped indentation where a bomb had dropped. They were old wounds of a horrible war, but here at Margraten was proof of the great price paid for peace.

Neatly trimmed grass offset the pure white marble crosses and occasional Star of David stones set in perfect symmetry. They seemed to gleam even in the face of the darkened sky. Most bore a name of the American soldier beneath. Some carried the inscription: "Here lies in honored glory a comrade in arms known but to God."

They lie not far from the battlefields in which they fell. I remembered a man back home telling me once about serving in an infantry regiment in this same general area. His had been nicknamed the diaper division because the soldiers were all under twenty-one. He shook his head as though to clear the insanity of it all as he remembered one company of these youths that had been completely wiped out.

That same old soldier, whom I was interviewing for an article for the local newspaper for Veteran's Day, had stopped at one point and covered his face with his hand. "I always prayed to the Lord." He told of long hours spent in foxholes. " 'If I can only get out of this mess and go home, that's all I want.' "

The marble walls we had rushed by near the reflection pool, we discovered, were inscribed with one thousand names of men whose bodies were never found. A tiny chapel nearby bore a prayer upon its wall: "O, Lord, Support us all the day long until the shadows lengthen and the evening comes and the fever of life is over and our work is done. Then in Thy mercy grant us a safe lodging and a holy rest and peace at last."

A paper from the visitor's building told how one headstone marked the common grave of two unknowns and that in no less than forty instances two brothers lie buried side by side.

I glanced at my nineteen-year-old son walking silently with me. Even our footsteps were hushed, as though the very ground was hallowed by the lives swept beneath. Forty-five years ago he might have been here, and one of these crosses could have been his.

The rain began with no fanfare of thunder or lightning. It simply fell softly and quietly like our tears. Inside, however, I felt as though a gully washer had just swept away my complacency and I would remember this place forever. I walked slowly back toward the car. Droplets of rain gathered on my hair, but it didn't seem important anymore.

> Father, I stretch my hands to Thee,
> No other help I know.
> If Thou withdraw Thyself from me,
> Ah, wither shall I go?
>
> CHARLES WESLEY

Everyone comes to a point in their life when an inner storm prevails and threatens to drown them with self-doubt. John Wesley recorded in his journal just such a time in his life. Eight months after what is known as his Aldersgate experience, where he was so moved by the Holy Spirit that he went on to establish the Methodist movement, he wrote the following journal entry:

> *My friends affirm I am mad because I said I was not a Christian a year ago. I affirm I am not a Christian now. For a Christian is one who has love, peace, joy. But these I have not. Though I have given, and do give, all my goods to feed the poor, I am not a Christian. Though I have endured hardship, though I have in all things denied myself and taken up my cross, I am not a Christian. My works are nothing. I have not the fruits of the Spirit of Christ. Though I have constantly used all means of grace for twenty years, I am not a Christian.*

Heroes of the Bible experienced inner storms, and their agony is recorded forever as they struggled to prevail.

Job—the patient one: "I call to you, O God,

but you never answer; and when I pray, you pay no attention" (Job 30:20 Good News Bible).

David—the beloved of God: "My God, my God, why have you abandoned me? I have cried desperately for help, but still it does not come" (Psalm 22:1 Good News Bible).

Solomon—the wise one: "God has laid a miserable fate upon us. I have seen everything done in this world, and I tell you, it is all useless. It is like chasing the wind" (Ecclesiastes 1:13–14 Good News Bible).

Paul (a saint): "For I know that nothing good dwells within me, that is, in my flesh. I can will what is right, but I cannot do it" (Romans 7:18 NRSV).

CORNERS

Adults aren't the only ones to endure inner storms. Children, too, struggle with right and wrong and lose out to life's temptations. My four-year-old grandson, Taylor, had been having a bad day. His unacceptable behavior finally reached his mother's last nerve, and he ended up standing in the corner for awhile.

As he stood there contemplating his shame

and guilt, his thoughts apparently rested on a higher giver of forgiveness than his mother. He knew he was already in big trouble with her or he wouldn't be studying the design on the wallpaper instead of playing with his friends.

He had always been full of questions. Who made the trees? Where did flowers come from? How did we get squirrels? Because he had seen pictures at Sunday school and had a simple concept of the man in them, his mother told him Jesus got the credit for all of that.

"Mama," Taylor's contrite voice could be heard from his place of punishment, "Jesus didn't make corners." Of course, she let him go. Who could hold such a thinker hostage?

There's a simple lesson to be gained by Taylor's insight. When we find ourselves cornered, we usually got there on our own. The wonderful part is that Jesus meets us there if we are willing, and there's no one better to have in your corner.

TROUBLED WATERS

Troubled waters flow,
restless,
over gravel-beds of worry,
second-guessing
what fate designed.

Hope walks
a slippery course,
crossing the bridges
in my mind.

AT THE WALL

On a day in late April, while Washington reveled in spring, a large group of sixth graders on a field trip and their chaperones stopped at the memorial wall that honors fallen soldiers of Vietnam. The children were too young to remember this time in history, but the adults did and felt sad and humbled at the sight of those gleaming panels.

Into this throng of sightseers rolled a man in a wheelchair. His fatigue jacket and patches identified him as a war veteran of that vintage.

He stopped and turned to study the names on a panel, then moved on to another. This appeared to be a pilgrimage as he scoured the names. Finally he found what he sought and made a sharp salute.

There is a guy who really belongs here, one observer thought to himself, *a man who has earned his stripes.* He wondered if the salute might have been for a long-ago comrade or maybe a commanding officer.

The old soldier wheeled himself back from the wall a short distance and sat there as if absorbed in thoughts of long-ago stormy battles. The man who had been watching him approached slowly. "Could I talk to you?" he asked softly.

"What do you want?" the soldier asked warily.

"Just to say thank you."

"For what?"

"For defending our country."

"What about all the others?" he asked as he inclined his head toward the memorial.

"Right now it's just you and me."

The soldier's demeanor softened. "No one's ever thanked me before," he said, and tears rolled down his face.

Sometimes just a kind word or a simple offering of thanks is all it takes to send a ray of sunshine into an inner storm.

THE TEDDY BEAR

Dennis is a Christian songwriter. The lyrics to his songs reflect his personal struggle to reach a place where he can write songs with titles such as "Christ Who Strengthens Me," "Who Am I?" or "I Need Some Repair." The childlike approach to his faith might seem simplistic as he sings one of his tunes like "Whisper in My Ear" or "On Jesus' Knee." His journey to reach the man he has become today who can pen these songs, however, is anything but simple.

This tall, rugged man is a recovering alcoholic. He knows firsthand the devastation of living in the throes of the ugly disease that robs its victims of dignity, sanity, and even their lives.

One of his songs tells of a teddy bear taken along on a camping trip. A storm blew in suddenly, and in the family's haste to leave, the hapless bear got left behind. Over time, fallen to the mercy of storms, he became covered with grime.

He remained lost and badly soiled until a stranger came one day and lifted him up from the debris. This stranger lovingly washed away the filth and held the little bear close to his heart. "That stranger was Jesus," his song ends, "and the teddy bear was me."

Shortly after he composed that tune, he happened to be driving through a rainstorm. In spite of the rain, something caught his eye near the side of the road. *Could it be?* he wondered as he found a place to turn his car around and head back. Sure enough, there in the downpour he plucked the soggy teddy bear from a puddle and wrung the muddy water from its body. Then this strapping man clutched the toy, and all that it represented to him, tight against his chest.

He carries it with him as he performs in churches throughout the area where he lives. It sits on one of the amplifiers, while he performs his music, as a reminder to him of where he has been and of the One who brought him out of the storm.

Let him have all your worries and cares,
for he is always thinking about you and
watching everything that concerns you.
Be careful—watch out for attacks from
Satan, your great enemy. He prowls
around like a hungry, roaring lion,
looking for some victim to tear apart.
Stand firm when he attacks. Trust
the Lord; and remember that other
Christians all around the world are
going through these sufferings too.

1 PETER 5:7–9 TLB

LESSON FROM A CHICKADEE

Fear. This inner storm causes us to react in various ways. It pumps adrenaline that gives us strength and speed for fight or flight. It can also paralyze, and both reactions can be life-savers. I realized one day, while watching birds at the feeder outside my front window, how wondrously equipped our Creator has made His creatures to weather life's storms.

Chickadees are my favorite bird. Besides his call that reminds me of a giggle, I love to watch this dapper little fellow at the feeder. He politely selects a sunflower seed and flits to a nearby tree, leaving the feeder free for others. There he hammers the seed between his beak and a branch until it pops open. This creates constant motion as each chickadee darts back and forth for every seed.

He is also the bravest bird at the feeder. All the others scurry with a fanfare of flapping wings when I approach, but not him. He sits barely inches away while I replenish his food supply and offers his jolly chick-a-dee-dee-dee as though he is singing for his supper.

I was so accustomed to his brisk behavior that it bewildered me one day when I looked out the window and saw a chickadee sitting at the feeder as though frozen, while a couple more sat motionless in the nearby cedar tree. I studied them, motionless myself, for several minutes as I tried to figure out why this tiny black-capped bundle of energy wasn't moving a feather.

Finally, as I glanced around for a clue to this puzzle, I noticed a large hawk perched near the top of a bare maple tree several yards away. That explained the chickadees' stillness. To panic and flee would mean disaster.

The line from Exodus 15:16 (KJV) probably wasn't penned with chickadees in mind, but it fit the occasion: "Fear and dread shall fall upon them; by the greatness of thine arm they shall be as still as a stone. . . ." Then again, I decided, why not? God must love the chickadee as much as I do. And who else would whisper in the storm, "Be still"?

I could take a lesson from my little bird friend. Too often, when trouble strikes, I become frantic. Mentally, emotionally, and sometimes physically, I run in circles when just a few minutes of stillness would serve me better. That is all it takes to place my fears of the storm in the care of the One who calms them.

FORGIVENESS

I have this notion of heaven
as a spotlessly clean,
freshly waxed floor,
stretching out before me,
while I stand at its edge
with muddy feet.

Right spirit.
Clean heart.
I pray for these
without a clear picture

of what I ask for.
Death to the old way,
rebirth of the new;
the child in me wonders,
will it hurt?

What price to be remolded?
What hard lessons
lead to obedience?
What will make me fit for heaven?

"Father, forgive them,"
Someone whispers.
And again, I have a notion
of a man
kneeling before His disciples,
tenderly
washing their feet.

BUMP IN THE NIGHT

Whenever I think of fear, my thoughts go back
to a summer night when I was thirteen. I had
been left in charge of my two little brothers for
the evening, and to sweeten the chore, Mom
had let me have a friend stay overnight.

A gentle breeze ruffled the curtains next to the bed where we lay talking and giggling over silly things young girls find so funny. My brothers were asleep in the next room. Something clattered loudly in the garage, which was several yards away from my open window.

"What was that?" my friend whispered. I suggested it might be our nearest neighbor, an eccentric old lady whom I figured might not be above prowling about in the moonlight. It was a plausible explanation, and my friend's deep, easy breathing soon told me I was the only one in the house who was still awake. Deep in my heart I knew our neighbor was slightly odd, but she wasn't crazy.

Then I heard it, the unmistakable snort of a black bear directly below my window. I was terrified. Afraid to move, lest I attract his attention, I barely allowed myself to breathe more than shallow breaths. My heart, however, hammered so loudly in my ears I worried the bear could hear it too. My mouth grew dry, and I don't think I could have screamed if my life had depended on it.

My mind, like my adrenaline-charged heart, worked overtime. I thought about the flimsy window screen and how it was all that stood between the bear and us. I pleaded with God to make that bear go away. How could I ever face Mom if I let my little brothers become part of the food chain?

After several minutes that dragged by like hours, I noticed the crickets starting to chirp again. I knew the bear had left. My parents returned soon after that. Mobilized at last, I met them at the door and sobbed uncontrollably.

Unlike my own children, I never thrilled to fright. No scary movies, haunted houses, or ghoulish costumes for me. I always chose something wimpy, like a cowgirl or princess getup for the Halloween party at school. Fear wasn't my forte.

Bible verses advising the faithful to fear God always bothered me. I found a lot of comfort in later versions that changed the word to "honor" or "revere." I figured the day-to-day storms of life were already fearful enough.

Trust Him when dark doubts assail thee,
Trust Him when trust is small,
Trust Him, when simply to trust Him
Is the hardest thing of all.

AUTHOR UNKNOWN

> *"I know you well—you are neither hot nor cold; I wish you were one or the other! But since you are merely luke-warm, I will spit you out of my mouth!"*
> REVELATION 3:15–16 TLB

HUCKLE-BUCKLE BEANSTALK

When a friend told me her relationship with God was like a game of huckle-buckle bean-stalk, she captured my attention. I had never heard of huckle-buckle beanstalk, but when she explained it, it sounded a lot like a game we played called hide-the-thimble.

The details of the game were simple. One person hid an object (could be a thimble) and guided the players to it by telling them if they were getting hot or cold, depending how close or far away they were.

My friend says the closer she comes to God and His will for her life, the warmer it is. When God seems distanced, she grows cold, like a dying ember removed from the fire. Her analogy gave me a lot to think about in my own relationship to God. Was I in danger of becoming lukewarm as the Scripture warned against? How do we move closer to God? I think we do it the same way we found the thimble when we were children. We make the effort. Pray. Search the Scriptures. Worship. Prepare for the storms that will surely come. If we do nothing, we are neither hot nor cold. In the game of huckle-buckle beanstalk, as well as the game of life, if we sit there like a luke-warm lump, we lose.

> *"I assure you that whoever does not receive the Kingdom of God like a child will never enter it."*
>
> MARK 10:15
> GOOD NEWS BIBLE

LIKE A CHILD

When my older son, Robby, was a small child, he had a deep fear of thunderstorms. He ran and hid from them whenever he could, but escape wasn't always possible. Sometimes he had to simply endure them. He reacted by squeezing his eyes tightly shut, hiding his face, and pressing his hands firmly over his ears. The best possible place, he learned, was on a safe, warm lap while being held in a tight hug.

I remember visiting friends at Fort Myers, Florida, when a thunderstorm blew in from the gulf. My grandmother happened to be on vacation with us, and she was one of Robby's favorite people. At the first roll of thunder, she quickly scooped her great-grandson up onto her lap and wrapped her arms around his tiny trembling body. They stayed that way all through the storm.

I guess because the emotions of raw fear and deep love were so strong at that moment, the mental image of the two of them has stayed with me all these years. Grandma has been gone for a long time, and Rob left that particular fear behind with his childhood.

I think, if we are acutely honest with ourselves, there remains a child inside us that still cries out for a safe lap when a bad storm brews. We may outgrow our fear of thunder and lightning, but there is always something that can shake us to our core.

As painful and scary as storms may be, however, they keep us moving. They move us to pray in a way the calm never can. They move us to think and take account of our lives. They move us to gratitude. They move us closer to our heavenly Father the same way we were prompted to find a safe lap when we were small. Somewhere in the heart of every storm, there is a child in need of a hug.

> *For I know the plans I have for you, says the Lord. They are plans for good and not for evil, to give you a future and a hope. In those days when you pray, I will listen. You will find me when you seek me, if you look for me in earnest.*
> JEREMIAH 29:11–13 TLB

VALLEY OF THE SHADOW

I didn't know him, but I felt the shock ripples when a teen in the community committed suicide. I wish someone could have shown him how to savor his existence before he reached that black pit where hope dies.

A sign in front of a church recently caught my eye. It read, "Evil turned around is Live," and it made me think again of that boy. I don't know what particular storm made him think his life had become so unbearable, but I know how it feels to live in that kind of despair and have thoughts of death dog your days. Fortunately for my family and me, I never went beyond the thinking and into the doing.

The darkness of that storm is so blinding it hides the bigger, brighter picture, but like the storm that can be measured in a rain gauge, life storms will pass. I wish I could have told the young man that no storm is worthy of your life, that he'd miss so many good gifts from God by not being there to accept them.

His suicide made me stop and take stock of just how much I would have missed if God had answered my prayer for Him to just let me die. I wouldn't have known my children as adults nor would I have been there to lend a helping hand when they needed me over the years. I would have missed that phone call from my daughter when she said, "You're going to be a grandma!" I would never have seen Europe, delivered a sermon, written a book, or fallen in love again.

The time span between that despairing prayer and today is filled with so many people I hadn't met yet who touched my life with goodness and joy. Of course, there have been a lot of storms too, but I wouldn't have wanted to miss them either. If there is one thing I've learned about God, it's that He likes walking in the rain.

I Believe

Does the Holy Ghost
go bump in the night,
scaring the little
fishhook-shaped question marks
into ramrod-straight,
exclamation-point
believers?

The highway is slippery,
and I have to drive.
Lord, I believe.
The highway is slippery,
and my teenager is driving
with my car,
and he's late.
Lord, help my unbelief.

A lump,
and the doctor says
we'll try this antibiotic
and see what happens.

Lord, I believe.
A lump,
and the doctor says
this is the name of a surgeon
he wants me to see.
Lord, help my unbelief.

A fire alarm
shatters the silence
of a late night's sleep
and quickens the beat
of a startled heart.
Lord, I believe.
Downstairs,
the front door slams
as my young volunteer fireman
responds to the call.
Lord, help my unbelief.

Sometimes it's all I have
in the night
when things go bump.

INNER STORMS PRAYER

Father God, thank You for Your presence that
penetrates the deep, scary places inside me
so I never have to go there alone.
By Your spirit, free me from obsessive
thinking that holds my mind hostage.
Help me to grow and learn from
my adversity. How could I give
compassion if I never knew pain?
How could I offer hope if I never felt despair?
How could I appreciate kindness if
I never experienced cruelty and indifference?
How could I impart wisdom if
I never stumbled on a pathway littered
with mistakes and wrong choices?
How could I fathom the full measure of
Your mercy and pardon if I deserved it?
Thank You, Lord, for these bitter life lessons
that cleanse the palate and
make me better able to savor joy.
Amen.

*Consider yourselves fortunate when all
kinds of trials come your way, for you
know that when your faith succeeds in
facing such trials, the result is the ability
to endure. Make sure that your endurance
carries you all the way without failing,
so that you may be perfect and complete,
lacking nothing. But if any of you lack
wisdom, you should pray to God, who
will give it to you; because God gives
generously and graciously to all. But
when you pray, you must believe and
not doubt at all. Whoever doubts is like a
wave in the sea that is driven and blown
about by the wind.*

JAMES 1:2–6
GOOD NEWS BIBLE

*Then in their trouble they called to the
Lord, and he saved them from their distress. He calmed the raging storm, and
the waves became quiet.*

PSALM 107:28–29
GOOD NEWS BIBLE

Stormy Relationships

God made us all wondrously different, and while that is a beautiful thing, it also creates an atmosphere for turbulence. Personalities clash with as much disturbance and surprise as a sudden hailstorm at a summer picnic where someone gets hurt.

Over and over in Scripture, the Bible urges us to be good to one another. In 1 Corinthians 1:10 (NIV) we find: "I appeal to you, brothers, in the name of our Lord Jesus Christ, that all of you agree with one another so that there may be no divisions among you and that you may be perfectly united in mind and thought." Again we hear it in 1 Peter 3:8–9 (NIV): "Live in harmony with one another; be sympathetic, love as brothers, be compassionate and humble. Do not repay evil with evil or insult with insult, but with blessing. . . ."

Ephesians 4:31–32 (NIV) advises us: "Get rid of all bitterness, rage and anger, brawling and slander, along with every form of malice. Be kind and compassionate to one another, forgiving each other, just as in Christ God forgave you." These letters to the early churches shape and guide us like a parent instructing a child.

It looks good on paper and sounds good in theory, but we become tangled in our emotions. Feelings are hurt, patience gets pushed to the breaking point, and we lose control until we don't even recognize ourselves in our behavior. Day-to-day living turns as scary and unpredictable as summer thunderstorms with a tornado watch. Pain is practically guaranteed when supercells with 100 percent chance of trouble move in.

Living together in peace and harmony takes effort as we come together in the world, our community, or at home. Storms happen, and it is at these times we question: Where is our faith?

The Chinese word for crisis is composed of two characters. The first stands for danger and the second for opportunity.

> *Be gentle and ready to forgive; never hold grudges. Remember, the Lord forgave you, so you must forgive others.*
> COLOSSIANS 3:13 TLB

Always remember. . . . Never forget. . . . Several inscriptions in my high school yearbook begin with these words. When they were penned I'm sure we thought these classes and adolescent escapades would burn in our memories forever. I find now, however, I can barely recall the classmates who wrote with such undying zeal, let alone the events.

Time has a way of winnowing our thoughts and leaving the oddest grains of memory behind. Miss Clark, for instance, will probably be a part of my high school recollections forever.

I had the strangest feeling she had gotten the job teaching at our school by mistake somehow. Surely, she would have fared better in a college where she would have been appreciated. She seemed to be older than most of the other teachers. Her thick glasses made her look like Mr. Magoo, and smeared mascara only confirmed the fact that she couldn't see much without them. Most of all, she appeared far too learned to bother with a class of silly teenage girls.

Tiny, scholarly, and gentle, she seemed an unlikely candidate to be at the center of a storm. I liked her, and I am embarrassed to admit, I kept that a secret. If anyone else in that class felt the same way I did, they kept quiet about it too. It was the outspoken ones who ruled. "We're not learning anything," they complained and took their grievances to the administration. They were persistent with their attack, while the rest of us said nothing in her defense. It took them only a few short months to win, and we found ourselves transferred to another class. I missed her terribly as I sat in the new room and diagrammed sentences.

Who cared that a statement could be rearranged like words swinging on a jungle gym? Miss Clark had challenged us to think and feel, and we had barely begun. It is hard to say how much we lost in that unfinished class, but for those few months, she lit a fire in my mind. She made famous writers come alive for me. Poet Sidney Lanier, languishing in prison as a captive soldier of the Civil War, became a real person as she talked. Guy de Maupassant, the writer whose name danced on the tongue; O. Henry, master of surprise endings; and Jack London, mighty adventurer, grew into authors worth reading.

Most of all, she led me to think. She

assigned a sentence for us to expand upon that became the last straw to her critics. They deemed it stupid and made the final complaint that got us moved. In a poetic bit of irony, they proved the truth of her assignment with their actions. She told us to write a short essay on the sentence: We are most easily attacked by that which we love most. Life would eventually teach all of us that pain was the price we sometimes have to pay for loving, but back then it was a truth yet unrevealed.

Her love and deep knowledge of literature, which she tried to impart to us, had lost her the class and brought her failure. I often wondered if she offered a defense. When we received our yearbooks at the end of the year, I ventured back to her room and asked her to sign mine. "Best wishes to a good pupil," she penned in flowing handwriting, "and a nice young girl."

Did she mean that? I wondered. How much did she perceive from behind those thick lenses? I was a part of that ungrateful class, my silence contributing to the shameful storm that hurt and humiliated her. Yet she rose above it and chose to forgive.

She left at the end of the year, and I never saw her again. I wish she could have known that in the midst of that cruel storm there was someone who would always remember and never forget what a wonderful teacher she had been.

SIDE STEPPER

I step cautiously,
Walking with happiness.
For she leads me
With a tapping cane
Down cobbled path stones
Of fragmented joys.
Where one misstep
Can sprain my heart.

LE STANTON

THE DAISY

I am a daisy.
He loves me.
He loves me not.

My petals are pulled away
one by one.
He loves me.
He loves me not.

What will the last petal say?
He loves me?
He loves me not?

By the time I know
If he loves me or not
I am torn apart.

Love's not gentle
To a daisy.

REBOUND

Here we are,
two casualties
from the battlefield
of romance.

Heart wounds
and pride bruises
abound.

Love and commitment
are locked tightly away
behind a door marked,
Never again.

Here we are,
two casualties.
Your kiss feels warm
against the loneliness.

*Future generations will serve him; they
will speak of the Lord to the coming
generation.*

PSALM 22:30
GOOD NEWS BIBLE

GENERATION GAP

"Where did I go wrong?" I silently demanded of rolling waves breaking onto the beach. I climbed one of the rocks exposed by low tide and stared at the wideness of the sea. I needed to remove myself from my two adolescent children before I said something I would regret or burst into tears.

When did I become my mom? I wondered. When had I arrived on the other side of the generation gap and become just like my mother? There wasn't anything wrong with Mom. It was the things I vowed never to say or do to my kids that I found myself saying and doing lately that smarted. Things my mother said. Things like "Where did I go wrong?"

"Father, help me," I implored, "everything feels out of control. I'm afraid for these children of mine who seem like strangers recently."

The three of us had decided to spend a few days at this seaside resort as a final summer getaway. Maybe this brief time away would magically erase the strain that had grown between my two younger children and me.

Leanne would start her senior year in high school next week. My relationship with my only daughter had been a tug-of-war lately. We couldn't manage to agree over much of anything. From clothes to curfew, we seemed to have drawn an invisible line in the sand and pulled our opposite ways. "You're my mother," she had told me one day in the middle of yet another disagreement. "I'm not supposed to agree with you." How could I win facing logic such as that?

Mark would head back to college in a couple weeks. He too, in a more subtle way, was turning into someone I didn't know anymore. There was the matter of the earring, which he knew I didn't like, that had quietly appeared while he was away at school.

"Oh, Lord, give me wisdom, strength, and patience," I prayed as I kept my back to the busy boardwalk and focused on the solitude of the sea.

This vacation that was supposed to be a bonding experience seemed to have exposed our differences instead. On the ride down, for instance, we couldn't agree on what music to play on the radio. Mine was too old-fashioned; theirs was too noisy.

Sharing a room wasn't easy either. I was a morning person; they were definitely nocturnal. When my energy shifted into reverse by late afternoon, theirs was ready for the fast lane.

This morning I had been awake since dawn. After three hours of reading, I felt hungry and eager to be on the beach. I opened the drapes, rattled a few suitcases, and finally ended up shaking them awake.

It turned out to be a case of leading the horse to water, or in this case, leading the teenagers to the beach. I could get them there but cooperation was something else. We walked on the boardwalk three abreast with me in the middle. I wanted to go down by the water and take some pictures. They flatly refused.

"My hair's a mess," Leanne complained.

"Later," Mark's clipped response agreed with his sister. No news here. Two against one; Mom's outvoted. Again.

Then the scene unfolded that sent me escaping to the rock. We noticed a maintenance man working on a ladder at a lamppost about ten feet ahead of us. As we approached, he lost his grip on a large ring of keys and it dropped with a clatter onto the boards. I automatically started forward with the intention of retrieving them.

Leanne jumped in front of me, however, grasped both my arms, and pushed me slightly backward. "What are you doing?" she demanded. "Are you crazy?"

I had been about to ask her the same thing. "That man's a total stranger," she continued. I could wrestle my teenage daughter to the ground and help the man or pass by on the other side like the bad guys in the Good Samaritan parable. Neither option appealed to me.

"You are too nice, Mom," Mark sided again with his younger sister, evidently taking my silence for submission rather than suppressed rage. He illustrated his point by saying it had taken us seven hours to make what he thought should have been a six-hour trip here because I wasn't an aggressive driver. Besides giving me something to think about the next time he wanted to borrow the car, his comment simply added fuel to an already slow burn inside me.

Fortunately for all of us, they spotted a shop with funky sunglasses and neat bathing suits and wanted to explore it further. I fled to the nearby rock to pout. I sat there, a newly initiated member of the older generation, and begged God to tell me where I had failed.

"What happened to the Golden Rule of doing unto others?" I inquired of a passing seagull as I replayed the incident with the dropped keys over in my mind. Was that concept as outdated as I felt at the moment?

I had never weathered a storm quite like this one before. My older son had eased through adolescence with few disturbances, leaving me unprepared for the turbulence of his younger siblings. I wish I could say we made that transition smoothly, but we didn't. Several years and prayer helped, however, and we survived without any storm-related casualties.

Not too long ago I had a conversation with Mark on one of his visits home. He told me about a man he met who was trying to travel around the world. Mark gave him a ride when it began to rain. When the man offered to sell him his sunglasses to raise some money for food, Mark refused. He gave him a little cash, however, and wished him well.

"You know, Mom," he confided, "sometimes I find myself saying or doing something, and I'll stop and think, 'That's just like my mother.' It's really strange."

I just smiled. Strange? Not at all. Welcome to the older generation, Son.

LETTING GO

I worry, here on the sideline,
As I watch this grown-up child of mine
Make mistakes.
For the babe I rocked secure and snug,
For a boy whose hurts I could fix with a hug,
My heart aches.

Life's answers, he'd seek then of me,
But now I feel cast as the enemy
And him a stranger.

I long to help, but don't know how.
How do you tell a big boy now,
Beware of danger?

Every word I say falls flat, off-key.
Each awkward step just shows that we
Don't understand each other.

It's funny, in some cosmic way,
Poetic justice, some might say,
But I've become my mother.

So Jesus called a child to come and stand in front of them, and said, "I assure you that unless you change and become like children, you will never enter the Kingdom of heaven. The greatest in the Kingdom of heaven is the one who humbles himself and becomes like this child. And whoever welcomes in my name one such child as this, welcomes me.

MATTHEW 18:2–5
GOOD NEWS BIBLE

NICOLE

Her name suggested a raven-haired beauty gracing pages of a romance novel with regal charm while dealing with life's drama and turmoil. Diaphanous gowns would fill her closet and declarations of undying love would fill her life.

I looked at the gangly, freckled child beside me and thought I knew why she responded more readily to Nicky.

Nicky and I met under a sad circumstance. At the moment we shared the room with a dead man who had been my uncle and her grandfather. A long procession of callers had hugged, kissed, and wept as they pressed through the dimly lit, flower-banked room. At its end, I had sunk gratefully into the nearest chair to relieve my tired feet rather than join the relatives in another room.

Nicky was the middle child of three sisters and tottered awkwardly on the edge of adolescence. Her older sister showed signs of emerging poise and beauty. I had noticed three teenage boys standing near her earlier, each apparently eager to console her.

The youngest sister was still a child. She would kneel at the rail near the casket and cry profusely, then, minutes later, attempt to master an acrobatic split just a few feet away.

Nicky had lagged behind too, seeming reluctant to leave. She cast a smile at me from the other side of the room and used it to reel herself into the seat next to mine. "I like that ponytail," I had told her earlier at our first encounter when I gave her hair a gentle tug. Her unruly brown mane had been pulled tightly to the side of her head with a rubber band and left to hang over her ear, creating a slightly lopsided effect. That simple gesture, it seemed, had won me her affection.

She was full of words, and they tumbled out freely. She wanted to talk about her grandfather and how she felt, how she had been told of his death but had intuitively known before her mother had said the words.

I asked about school; was it finished for the summer? No, she had another week to go, and she would be in the sixth grade next fall. She was eleven years old, she said.

"My mother and father are still married," she volunteered unexpectedly, "but they don't live together."

"I told my father about Grandpa dying and asked him to come here tonight," she confided, "and he said he would try." Was that why she still lingered, I wondered, in the slim hope that he would come, that a promise to his daughter meant something important to him?

She admitted he wouldn't be particularly welcomed by his wife's family, and I felt sorry for this child caught in the middle of an adult war.

"I'm afraid my dad will die," Nicky confessed while her eyes filled with tears. "He's the only man left now." She had her mother, sisters, grandmother, and aunts. Her grandfather, I gathered, had been the one man in her life who paid any attention to her. A bad father, she had decided, was better than no father at all.

It was time to go. I hugged the skinny child, and we exchanged kisses as we vowed to see each other at the next family reunion. My first thoughts had been wrong, I realized; this girl knew more than she should about life's drama and turmoil.

"Good-bye," she said with a brief wave of her hand.

I lifted my hand almost as a benediction. "Good-bye, Nicole." May God be with you.

Accept one another, then, for the glory of God, as Christ has accepted you.
ROMANS 15:7
GOOD NEWS BIBLE

THE AGAPE MEAL

It is difficult when storm clouds engulf a relationship, and it is especially hard when it happens in a church. That old joke about the minister who pleased 100 percent of his congregation—half when he came and half when he left—didn't seem quite so funny when it actually happened.

That was the situation the committee in charge of the agape meal found themselves in on that Maundy Thursday night. They had worked hard at preparing foods with symbolic meaning, hoping they would create a sense of reality and appreciation for the night Jesus was betrayed.

Now, as the greens wilted and the baskets of dried fruits and nuts sat untouched, the only reality they faced was that no one was coming.

It was 1972 and war raged in Vietnam while protesters sported peace signs in an effort to make their feelings known. When the new minister let his hair grow longer than some thought proper, wore an occasional peace sign, and took a stand on the side of peace, the upheaval on a global level personalized within their small-town church. Unkind words were hurled until longtime friends no longer spoke to each other.

Boycotting the agape meal, however, came as a surprise to the ones who had planned it. As they looked at the empty places at the long table they had prepared with a white tablecloth and rustic candles, the rejection became tangible. They felt deeply hurt.

There were about a dozen people, counting committee members and spouses, and they paced and glanced often at the door that remained sadly shut. When it became obvious it was too late, even for stragglers, the minister suggested a bold idea.

He knew of a bus that had broken down on the interstate highway that ran beside their town. It sat in a garage near the church, and maybe, just maybe, the stranded passengers would welcome the fellowship and simple meal of fish and unleavened bread. The minister and two of the men went to offer the invitation while the rest waited to see what this small step of faith would produce.

A rock group, it turned out, owned the bus, and they had been experiencing their own share of rejection that day. It was bad enough to have mechanical problems, but they were also stuck in a small country town where they were not welcomed. Their long hair, fringed vests, and bell-bottoms made them a target of suspicion. Even the local shopkeepers treated them coolly. When they were approached by the three men with a friendly offer to attend their agape meal, they quickly accepted.

They made an unusual group when everyone was finally seated at the table. Ironically, the young musicians filled the exact number of empty places. As conversation commenced, the hosts learned the men were from Ohio and were on their way home after spending some time in New York City making a record. When someone offered to run home for the groceries to make a more substantial meal, their guests refused. This was just fine, they insisted; in fact, it was wonderful. Everyone ate the tuna fish and pita bread and munched on dates and figs and dried apples as happily as if it were fine dining.

After the meal, the minister invited them to the sanctuary for a brief worship service and communion. Pearls and love beads, bell-bottoms and dress slacks, the two groups kneeled as one to share the common cup. Afterwards the men asked if they could sing for their new acquaintances.

First they sang "We'll Get By with a Little Help from Our Friends," then one of the men shared a love song he had just written. It was so new he had to sing without music, but his clear, strong voice filled the sanctuary and gave everyone goose bumps.

Thank-yous, hugs, and tears marked their farewell, and the two groups were left with a lot to ponder that night. Agape is a Greek word meaning love, but it is a special kind of love. God's love for man, the dictionary defines it, spontaneous and unselfish. There in the middle of a storm of hate and rejection they had experienced agape, the purest love of all.

Talk with Me

Talk with me,
make a pathway of words
that I may follow inside
and know you better.

Talk with me,
let me paint a self-portrait
with my thoughts
upon your mind and heart.

Talk with me,
tell what you believe,
and how you feel
and where your hopes are bound.

Find a common ground
where likeness stands
and bridges our differences.

Talk with me
before it's too late.

Lord God, forgive us, please,
for the measure of miserableness we inflict
upon each other. We have wonderful
intentions of cruising through life in harmony
with each other, but we keep getting jolted
by life's speed bumps along the way.
Instill in us, we pray, a kinder spirit
when we disagree and a forgiving nature
when we've felt the pain of unfairness.
Teach us what to do with our anger when it
threatens to bubble over into destructive rage.
Guide us, Lord, through the storm-tossed days
when it's hard to keep afloat. Just as You
smoothed the waters on the Sea of Galilee,
still wrong intentions in such as we.
Amen.

STORMY RELATIONSHIPS PRAYER

*Father, we know You love each and
every one of Your children.
At least, that Sunday school concept
sits deep in our memory files.
Forgive us, Lord, but unconditional love
is not a simple concept to grasp.
We're tempted to point out the unfair acts
against us and wonder how heaven's mercy
can extend to someone who obviously
doesn't deserve it.
Then we are reminded by some still,
small voice inside us that we, too,
are undeserving in many ways.
Help us to forgive our sisters and brothers,
Father, as we now ask that grace
for ourselves as well.*

Amen.

Sudden Storms

Sudden storms strike without warning and bring a flashflood of trouble. A telephone rings, brakes squeal, or a split-second wrong decision and our world is swept out of our hands.

Like the disciples caught in the sudden squall on the lake, we react with raw emotion. Panic, fear, or grief overwhelms us, and we can barely formulate a prayer beyond a desperate cry of help.

Sometimes they appear in life-and-death drama and other times they loose their turbulence within us. Even in this kind of storm, however, the Lord still calls, "Where is your faith?" Grab hold of your faith and hold on until the storm is gone.

So now there are pitfalls all around you, and suddenly you are full of fear. It has grown so dark that you cannot see, and a flood overwhelms you.

Job 22:10–11
Good News Bible

I realized another thing, that in this world fast runners do not always win the races, and the brave do not always win the battles. The wise do not always earn a living, intelligent people do not always get rich, and capable people do not always rise to high positions. Bad luck happens to everyone. You never know when your time is coming. Like birds suddenly caught in a trap, like fish caught in a net, we are trapped at some evil moment when we least expect it.

ECCLESIASTES 9:11–12
GOOD NEWS BIBLE

COPPERHEAD

"Stop! It's a snake," someone yelled when the headlights exposed a copperhead stretched across the warm pavement. Three teenage boys bounded from the car on a reckless mission of making the world a little safer.

With the dubious invincibility of youth, they ignored the fact that they had no means to kill the creature and were clad only in wet bathing suits and sneakers. No one thought of simply running the car's wheel over the snake. This was primal. This was war. This was mob mentality, peer pressure, and foolishness combined to make conditions ripe for a storm of dangerous proportions.

The trio had been for a midnight swim, and the mood was one of excitement and daring. Someone quickly rummaged through the car for a weapon and came up with the unlikely combination of a plastic ice scraper and a beach towel.

The snake was the only one to respond to the situation sensibly. He attempted to crawl away. This heightened the adrenaline, and one of the boys tossed sand in the serpent's eyes to stop him.

A second youth threw the beach towel over the agitated snake and pinned his head against the pavement with the ice scraper, causing the rest of its body to writhe in protest. "Pick him up," someone dared Kevin, the remaining boy.

"I don't like this," Kevin responded as he reached for the extremely irritated snake. The fire that rushed through his hand as the flimsy scraper slipped and the snake sank its fangs deep into his flesh made the young man think this must be what it feels like to grab hold of a live 220-volt wire.

A normal copperhead bite consists of a quick strike, release, and retreat. This creature, however, was so frenzied he continued to hang on, emptying his poison sacks until Kevin managed to pull him off with his other hand.

The swelling began immediately as three badly frightened teens debated what to do first. After failing to find the family doctor at his home, they drove on to the emergency room. Ill-equipped to handle an affliction of this sort, the doctor on call at the small facility fumbled with the directions on a snake bite kit while someone called the police for an escort to a larger hospital fifteen miles away.

Someone else contacted Kevin's mother, and she arrived just as two troopers were preparing to take her son in the police car. "I'm going to give your mother a ticket," the younger officer complained to Kevin as they raced with flashing lights and blaring siren with her staying tight to their tail.

"No," his older partner countered, "she's just being a mother."

The fangs had entered the muscle between his thumb and pointer finger. After the initial sensation of liquid fire in his veins, the pain subsided some. The swelling continued to spread to his whole hand and started up his arm. The first thing they did at the larger hospital was cut his class ring to remove it.

Kevin had worked part-time pumping gas all summer. Constant exposure to gasoline toughens the skin, and this made it difficult to insert the needle to start the intravenous. The pain was increasing, and he felt as though he was on fire.

"You have to make a decision right now," a doctor told him. "I have to give you injections of horse serum. Do you want 1000cc in each buttock or 10cc in each eyeball?"

Kevin rolled over, pulled down his wet bathing suit, and said, "Have at it."

"I've got to do some work on your hand," the doctor continued, "but I can't give you anesthesia because the bite is too close to your heart." Five orderlies appeared quickly at his side and gripped each leg, arm, and his head while the doctor cut away at the damaged flesh.

Kevin screamed until he finally passed out from the pain. When he regained consciousness, he was in intensive care. His arm was black and the swelling had nearly climbed to his shoulder. Doctors were prepared to amputate his arm if it went any farther. His feverish body lay packed in ice. He had never been so afraid in his life nor had he ever prayed so hard.

He awoke again to see a priest standing over him giving him last rites. "You know, Father," he said, "I'm not Catholic."

"I know," answered the man of God.

"Oh, God, I don't want to die yet," the young man cried as he drifted again into oblivion.

Kevin's storm happened nearly thirty years ago. A small white scar near his thumb is all the visible reminder he has of that time. A popular theory suggests a coincidence is a small miracle where God chooses to remain anonymous. Kevin's story has just such an element to it.

A snake hunter had been bitten by a rattlesnake one week before Kevin's encounter with the copperhead. He was taken to the same emergency room and found the staff unprepared to treat his problem. He, however, was well equipped to handle the situation, having been bitten a few times before. He carefully instructed the doctor on what to do. The incident bothered the doctor so much, he researched the treatment of snake bites all week until he became quite knowledgeable on the subject.

Of all the doctors on the staff at that large hospital, he was the one on call the night Kevin came in, the only doctor who knew what to do.

Protect me, Lord, from the power of the wicked; keep me safe from violent people who plot my downfall.

PSALM 140:4
GOOD NEWS BIBLE

ANGEL IN A DERBY

Donna's storm struck suddenly, without warning and with the capability to destroy. She was eighteen and worked as a clerk at a city hospital. One night a week she had to stay until nine o'clock, when visiting hours ended. She liked working during the daytime better, when the large waiting area bustled with patients coming for clinics and lab work. Sitting at a desk in the isolated corridor and handing out visitor passes felt spooky, especially with the darkened examining rooms that lined both sides of an empty hall.

There were always stragglers after visiting hours ended, and this made her late closing up. She stood at the tall desk, putting the last of the passes in order, when she realized someone had come up behind her. "Oh, Doctor," she exclaimed when she recognized the man standing so close she could hear his breathing, "what are you doing here?"

Ignoring her question, the intern reached for her left arm and twisted it behind her back. "You're coming with me," he ordered as he pushed her around the desk and down the long, dimly lit waiting area.

"Wh–where?" she stammered as panic tightened her throat.

He wasn't a large man, but he had a stocky build. At barely five feet tall and weighing only ninety-three pounds, she was no match for his strength. He had always made her feel uncomfortable with his flirting and comments about how cute she looked. Besides, he was a married man.

"Let me go. Let me go!" she pleaded, but

he just tightened his grip on her twisted arm and shoved her along faster.

A small hallway led off the end of the waiting area; he pushed her around the corner and down the short corridor. Two small restrooms were on the left and a utility room where the outpatient nurses stored supplies occupied the right.

He stopped near the utility room door and backed her against the wall, still keeping her left arm bent against her back and her right arm pinned to her side. "We're going in here and have some fun," he said as he pressed his body against hers and tried to kiss her.

She struggled, turning her face away from his. "If you don't let me go," she cried, "I'm going to scream."

"Who's going to hear you?" he responded with a laugh.

"You can't do this," she insisted. "I'll tell everybody."

"Who'd believe you?" he sneered, and she feared he was probably right. He was a doctor. She was just a teenaged girl.

He forced her slowly toward the door in spite of her resistance until a sudden light cut across the dim hallway and fell upon them.

The door to the men's restroom stood wide open and a man framed the doorway with light spilling around him. Attired in a long, black dress coat and a black derby hat, he looked the epitome of a dignified gentleman, a stark contrast to the scene before him. His eyes fixed on the couple, but he did not speak or move.

The doctor quickly released his grip and fled, leaving Donna slumped against the wall. With a polite nod of his head, the stately stranger walked past her and around the corner.

Where had he come from? she wondered. She would have seen him walk past her desk, especially someone as striking as he. She ran after him to pour out her gratitude, but the whole waiting area was empty. He couldn't have reached the door that quickly, but he had vanished as mysteriously as he appeared. Her ready words of thanks died on her lips and settled somewhere in her heart as a humble prayer. The storm was over as quickly as it began, and she had no doubt who had stopped its violent course.

LAST GIFT FOR GRANDMA

The phone call wasn't unexpected. I knew my grandmother was dying. She had, in fact, asked me to pray for her to die the last time I saw her only days before. The quality of her life had slipped to nil as she struggled with illness and infirmity. No one who loved her could selfishly wish to hold her back while heaven waited. Still, when my aunt called and said, "Grandma's gone," a storm of grief claimed me.

Perhaps because I had been her first granddaughter and lived next door, she and I had a close bond. She could make me feel valued in a way no one else ever did. Childhood memories of her patiently indulging my little girl whims flooded my mind after I replaced the receiver.

She let me use her kitchen to concoct outlandish dishes to feed her cats, then cleaned up the mess. Grandma never objected when I tugged at her apron strings and pretended she was my horse in a harness while she calmly worked about the house.

I thought about a long bus trip to New York City with Grandma to see the circus and how we bought lunch at the automat. This was a new experience for her too, and like a kid in a candy shop, she selected all desserts. When someone to whom you were special is gone, I wondered, do you stop being special?

I cried. Grieving exacted it. After that initial reaction, however, I focused on something else my aunt had said. Would I write a poem for Grandma's funeral? I told her I would try but wondered how I could focus on writing when my heart was breaking.

Later that evening after the rest of my family had gone to bed, I sat on the floor in front of the glowing remnants in the fireplace and began to write. As words began to shape sentences and create images, I could feel the icy grip of grief thaw a little.

When I finished, I had written not only a poem, but also a short essay about her life. I wanted the minister to know more about her so he would be able to eulogize someone other than the sick elderly lady he had called upon. Maybe I could give him a more rounded picture of the person she had been. I told of the young woman who whimsically sent away for the army surplus parachute, which provided my cousins and me with yards and yards of white silk to play dress-up. I presented a glimpse of the daring lady who talked me into taking a helicopter ride with her over Niagara Falls. I white-knuckled the seat while she delighted in the thrill of the adventure.

On the day of her funeral the minister was delayed and arrived just in time to begin the service. He quickly stepped to the lectern, fumbled with his papers, and proceeded to read my words. All of them. Without meaning to, I wrote the final tribute to Grandma. A parting gift, a public pronouncement of the wonderful humanness of her life, helped me through that last good-bye. I think she would have liked it that way.

SAYING GOOD-BYE TO GRANDMA

Do you have to go already?
she'd ask
when it was time to go away.

Well, what's your hurry?
was her appeal to us
to stay.

Stay and eat,
she'd hasten to oblige
with a table quickly set.

Baked beans are in the oven,
but the potatoes
have a bone in 'em yet.

Hair net and homemade apron,
potted plants and old porch swing—
always there, ever steady.

We, the wounded,
Bring you flowers, Grandma.
Do you have to go already?

SUDDEN STORMS PRAYER

*God, our Sustainer, watch over us,
we pray, when trouble strikes so
unexpectedly it sweeps our defenses away.
Hear our desperate plea,
please, and have mercy upon us.*
Amen.

LIFE-CHANGING STORMS

In the eye of a hurricane, the path of a twister, or the grip of a blizzard we fear for our lives. There are human events that equal these cataclysmic acts of nature and threaten our existence too. Birth, living, and death all hold pitfalls that shake us to our marrow and make us question our existence and whether we can endure another minute of it.

A storm, especially a violent one, makes us feel small and vulnerable. The terror and helplessness we experience reinforces the fact that we are not in command of our environment and that life is fragile.

When faced with these forces beyond our control, faith is our surest way to survival. The effort to reach out for that lifeline isn't always easy. Sometimes it seems beyond our grasp, but we are required only to reach. The One who reaches back simply asks, "Where is your faith?" not how strong it is.

For I am certain that nothing can separate us from his love: neither death nor life, neither angels nor other heavenly rulers or powers, neither the present nor the future, neither the world above nor the world below. . . .

ROMANS 8:38–39
GOOD NEWS BIBLE

OUT OF THE BLUE

One of the things Jerry liked best about being an airplane pilot was rising above the clouds into what he reverently called God's Terrain or God's Space. He never failed to be humbled when he entered that silent, pristine world of blue sky and sunshine where peace and beauty graced his soul. It always prompted a prayer of gratitude to feel so close to the Creator. The Twenty-third Psalm came often to mind in a setting such as this. No matter how much it might storm on the ground, he knew that five minutes after takeoff would find him above all the bad weather.

For twenty-five years he met God in the sky, and it seemed to him they flew together over the top of life's storms as well as around the occasional thunderstorm cell. Then he awoke one morning in a hotel room in Lakeland,

Florida, to discover his life had been forever grounded. God's Terrain at the top of fluffy white clouds was no longer within his reach.

He had just finished his annual week of intense training where, with the help of a simulator, pilots faced more emergency situations in a few days than they could expect in ten lifetimes. No simulator in the world, however, could have prepared Jerry for the storm of trouble that was about to change his life.

The digital clock showed 4:30 A.M., too early to get up yet. In a few hours he would take a limousine to Tampa to catch a flight for Pittsburgh, Pennsylvania, then on to Harrisburg, where his wife would meet him for the drive home to York.

He felt uncomfortably warm. Feverish, he decided, as he touched the back of his hand to his forehead. A couple of aspirin should help. Swinging his feet over the side of the bed, he stood and immediately collapsed in a heap on the floor. Three times he tried to stand, and three times he slammed back onto the floor.

"This can't be happening to me," he declared to the darkened room. "Oh, God, please help me."

As Jerry lay there trying to make sense of

this terrible situation, he knew what he must do. Cold water would bring his fever down. He began a slow, wobbly crawl into the bathroom, where he turned on the cold water and pulled himself into the tub. After about fifteen minutes, his fever vanished, and he had his equilibrium back.

By the time he reached Pittsburgh, however, he walked with a stagger. He clung to a handrail to keep from falling and knew from the disapproving looks of other travelers that they thought he was drunk. Jerry had never felt so alone or frightened in his life. *What is happening to me?* he despaired. He was a lone island of misery in normal, everyday surroundings with people going about their business. How had he awakened into the twilight zone?

By the time his wife drove him home from Harrisburg, he slurred his speech and had trouble concentrating. She called an ambulance.

After a battery of tests and consultations, the diagnosis sounded a death knell to his career. Multiple sclerosis. They might as well have pronounced him dead, he felt; no more venturing into God's Terrain for him. His wings were clipped forever.

"I have a piece of advice I'd like to give you," one of his doctors offered after awhile. He suggested Jerry acquire a pool membership and swim every morning.

Where do you go when God's in His heaven but nothing is right in your world anymore? What do you do when you feel so storm-battered that you will never be the same again? Swimming didn't seem like much, but it was something. "What do I have to lose?" he responded halfheartedly.

That first morning he approached the pool and slowly eased himself into the water until ripples lapped at his waist. He stood there for awhile then lunged into a swim. Chlorine stung his nose and his strokes were labored.

The Twenty-third Psalm came unbidden into Jerry's thoughts. *The Lord is my shepherd,* the words began in his mind, *I shall not want. He leads me beside still waters* seemed especially appropriate at the moment. *He restores my soul* and *Thou art with me* felt like a prayer.

It took an hour to swim forty laps, which was equal to one nautical mile. Day after day and mile after mile he swam and prayed. It grew to be such an important part of his day that Jerry found he would rather miss eating than to interrupt that hour he spent in the water talking with God.

He kept a record of his mileage by highlighting his progress on one of his old aviation charts with a felt-tipped marker. He swam the federal airways he used to fly. It took him four and one-half years to complete one thousand miles. His laps in the pool equaled the route he used to fly from Thomasville, Pennsylvania, to Fort Myers, Florida.

"Now that I'm down here, what must I do?" Jerry wondered aloud as he stared at the bright pink line on his map. "You swam down here," came the words firmly imprinted across his mind, "swim home. Rely on My strength and not yours."

In spite of missed time with heart surgery, Jerry's highlighted route finally made it back home. What used to take six and one-half to eight hours' flying time to go to Florida and back, took him nearly six years to swim.

Jerry continued to set goals, swimming enough laps to equal 150 nautical miles to his high school reunion, then on toward the New England states, where an old air force buddy lived. Crossing the Canadian border proved too irresistible, so he logged enough laps to make it to Ottawa.

By the end of the year 2000 he marked the four-thousand-mile mark of his morning swims. Twelve years after his diagnosis, he is still mobile. His doctor at Hershey Medical uses Jerry as an example to others who are stricken with that disease.

As vital as that swimming pool has become to the quality of his life, the real driving force for Jerry is his Lord, who stays there with him. Their relationship above the clouds was special, but it is God's presence into the storm clouds and beyond that keeps Jerry going. No matter where he goes, now he knows he is always in God's Terrain.

> *We do not live to ourselves, and we do not die to ourselves. If we live, we live to the Lord, and if we die, we die to the Lord; so then, whether we live or whether we die, we are the Lord's. For to this end Christ died and lived again, so that he might be Lord of both the dead and the living.*
>
> ROMANS 14:7–9 NRSV

Judy was headed for trouble. She had fallen in with the wrong crowd, a group of older kids who seemed bent on destruction. Then she became pregnant at fifteen and learned to grow up in a hurry.

Abortion, she decided, was not an option, and when she learned she was carrying a boy, she decided to keep him. She was the oldest of four sisters and liked the idea of having a boy in the family.

Justin came two months early by cesarean section when the doctor found he had stopped growing. He weighed barely four pounds, and doctors believed he had suffered a stroke while in the womb. His left side didn't develop as quickly or as well as his right, causing him to limp as he grew older.

Health problems continued to plague the tiny boy, starting with a series of ear infections and then pneumonia when he was two. After several bouts of pneumonia, he was diagnosed at age four with a disease that caused his blood count to fluctuate. A port was placed in his side, whereby he received monthly doses of gamma globulin. He seemed to improve.

Small and sickly, the little boy depended more than usual upon his mother, and she didn't let him down. Though she wasn't many years beyond babyhood herself, she handled the responsibility. She missed a lot of school, but with cooperation from the system, she managed to earn respectable grades. Whenever she got a rare night out, she was always the designated driver because she couldn't bare the thought of anything happening to her and leaving Justin without a mother. Judy even learned to give her son his medication, including injections and caring for the port in his side, because Justin didn't want anyone else to do it.

She graduated, found employment, and she and Justin got a place of their own. She met Tim, and they planned to marry. Justin seemed to like the idea. Then when Justin was seven, she faced a storm far greater than anything she had ever known.

She noticed his stomach was swollen, and she took him to the emergency room. His liver was enlarged, they told her, possibly from hepatitis. An ultrasound showed spots on his liver and kidneys. A biopsy brought the shattering news that it was cancer.

Judy and Tim had planned a May wedding,

but as Justin grew sicker from the chemotherapy, they decided to wait. They simply couldn't be married without their ring bearer.

Justin developed mouth sores from the chemo and ate very little. His tiny thirty-two-pound body lost ten more pounds. They spent a lot of time at the hospital, and Judy appreciated the nurses' caring and kind manner to both Justin and her. They watched her help with her son and told her she should go to nursing school.

The day the doctor told them of Justin's cancer, Judy went upstairs with her mother and sat on the edge of a bed. "What's going to happen if he dies?" she asked. Her mother assured her everything would be all right, but deep down the horrible thought wouldn't go away. What happens if he doesn't make it?

She felt angry. Everyone in her family was praying for Justin, but she couldn't bring herself to talk to the God who would let her son suffer so, except to occasionally ask, "Why aren't You doing anything?"

Judy and Tim married on June 7, and Justin was the ring bearer, as planned, but his grandmother had to carry him down the aisle. The newlyweds went away just overnight and, for the first time, Justin cried when she left him.

About once a week, Judy would break down and cry uncontrollably. It was evident that Justin was losing his battle with the disease. She and her mother were in a break room at the hospital when she lost control and began to sob. "We need to pray that God either heals him or takes him home," her mother said, and Judy had to admit she was right.

A couple of weeks later, Judy stopped on her way home from work to pick Justin up at her mother's house, where he had spent the night before. "Are you ready?" she asked him as he lay on his grandmother's bed, and he answered, "No, not yet."

They lived just a couple of minutes away, and she told him she was going home to straighten things up a bit. There wasn't much to do, however, because she had given Justin's room a thorough cleaning the day before. In about fifteen minutes, her mother called and said Justin wanted her.

When he saw his mother, he said, "Mama, I'm ready to go home." They were his last words. She felt his body go limp in her arms and, laying him on her mother's lap, dialed 911.

In the emergency room they began CPR

and gave him medicine to restart his heart. His frail body was connected to so many tubes, and when Judy asked about the bleeding from his mouth, they told her it was probably from his lungs.

She felt faint with shock, fear, and an overwhelming guilt. She should have known, her dazed mind insisted as it grabbed for some form of control. If only she had brought him to the hospital earlier. As Tim led her from the room, she began to scream, "It's my fault."

Justin was admitted to intensive care, and the doctor told Judy there was nothing more they could do. He asked if she wanted them to restart his heart again if needed. He had suffered enough, she realized, and told the doctor no.

When it was over and his tiny heart finally put his body to rest, they allowed his family back into the room. They gathered in a circle and each told Justin whatever was on their mind. Then Judy asked to be left alone with her son. With tears streaming down her face, she held him and told him how sorry she was that this had happened. She reminisced of their brief life together and wondered aloud what she was going to do without him. Most of all, she told him how much she loved him. For over an hour she cried and talked until her mother came in and said, "It's time to go."

"It's so hard," Judy uttered as she walked away without looking back.

"I know," her mother answered, "but he's in a better place now." It wasn't what Judy wanted to hear.

When she got home she went directly to his room. She wanted something that still held his smell. She reached for his pillow but put it back. She had laundered it the day before. Then her gaze fell on the baseball cap he had worn when his hair fell out from the chemo treatments. His head had been so small, her mother had cut and resewn the back so it would fit. She spent the night there among his things, hugging the baseball cap that smelled like her little boy, and mourned his loss.

His tombstone bears the inscription across the top: "Seven years of heaven here on earth." On the bottom is the answer to the little prayer she and her mother uttered two weeks before he died: "He is healed now."

An autopsy revealed the chemotherapy had rid him of the cancer, and a virus had attacked his weakened body. There was nothing more his mother could have done for him. Eventually the guilt and anger went away, but she still thinks of him every day.

"There's no telling where I'd be if I hadn't gotten pregnant," Judy says today of her life with Justin. "I might be into drugs or alcohol." Today it is prescription drugs and rubbing alcohol that fill her thoughts as she studies hard to become a nurse. She wants to work in pediatrics.

"I've been through what those parents are going through now," she says. "I want to make a difference in someone else's life for Justin. I don't want him to have lived and died in vain."

NOT FAIR

We lived on a dead-end street in a small town. Little traffic and sprawling backyards made it a good place to raise children. There was always a game of some sort going on with several of the neighborhood kids. Then they grew up and went on to other things and the street grew quieter, as though it daydreamed of childish laughter.

Cathy was a small child when her parents built the house across the street from us. We saw her grow into a coltish young girl and then into a young woman. She became a nurse, specializing in trauma and rescue, and was engaged to a young man also involved with air rescue.

A two-word headline in the local newspaper, "Coptcr Crashes," shattered the quiet of our little street and plunged her parents into the worst storm of their lives. Cathy, her patient, and the pilot were all killed when the helicopter in which they were flying crashed into the side of a mountain. She lost her life doing the work she loved. The following is a poem I wrote for her memorial service:

> A flick
> of fate's finger,
> and our world turns topsy-turvy
> like Lilliputian children
> or counterpane soldiers
> flung by a mighty
> undiscerning force.
>
> It's not fair,
> a grieving mother sobs.
> She wants her child back
> and we can offer only
> hugs and coffee cake.

No, it's not fair, we agree,
Her daughter was on a mission of mercy,
a community servant.
Why didn't death lick its hungry lips
over a drug dealer on the street corner
instead.
It's not fair,
my neighbor cries
as I hold her close and mumble,
"If there's anything I can do. . ."

Cathy's parents established a scholarship fund in her memory at the college where she had graduated. So far, it has helped three young women, chosen by the college, who were four-year nursing students in dire need of financial assistance. They each received money every semester to cover tuition and expenses.

Cathy's mother describes the first student chosen as "a bubbly personality like Cathy," and that helped ease some of the pain.

Out of this tragic storm, a young woman's dream lives on in the lives of others who reach for the same star.

*Heavenly Father, we turn to You,
too numb with grief to offer a coherent
prayer beyond Oh, God...Oh, God....
We feel broken beyond repair. Hold us
close, we pray, and grant us Your peace,
strength, and abiding love to ride out this
storm that feels like it will never end.*
                                    Amen.

*And in the same way—by our faith—the
Holy Spirit helps us with our daily problems and in our praying. For we don't
even know what we should pray for, nor
how to pray as we should; but the Holy
Spirit prays for us with such feeling that
it cannot be expressed in words. And the
Father who knows all hearts knows, of
course, what the Spirit is saying as he
pleads for us in harmony with God's own
will. And we know that all that happens
to us is working for our good if we love
God and are fitting into his plans.*
                          ROMANS 8:26–28 TLB

*Hope in the LORD! For with the LORD
there is steadfast love, and with him is
great power to redeem.*

PSALM 130:7 NRSV

HER ONLY SON

Leta didn't suspect she might be pregnant until a doctor delivered the stunning news when she was already five months into the pregnancy. She knew a girl who had faced a similar situation a few months before and handled it with an abortion. When she asked about the same solution for her, the doctor told her she was too far along for that. Today she thanks God for keeping her from doing something she feels she would have regretted the rest of her life.

She had recently lost the young man she had dated steadily for three years when he was killed. A brief fling, perhaps on the rebound from her loss, resulted in the unwanted circumstances. She was twenty, had a good job, and was paying for a car. She also led an active church life.

Her mother's stance was, "Look what

you've done to me." To avoid embarrassment to her family in Alabama, she was sent to live with her brother and sister-in-law on the West Coast.

No one ever suggested she keep the baby or offered to help her if she did. She knew from the onset that she would have to give the child away. That knowledge didn't lessen the feelings growing inside her heart as surely as the fetus grew inside her womb. Sometimes she gave in to these yearnings and spread her hands across her swelling abdomen. That was as close as she could come to holding her unborn child as she cried and whispered, "I don't want to give up my baby."

Her brother and sister-in-law were kind to her, and she attended church with them. Her sister-in-law was due to give birth about a month before Leta.

She worried how she would be able to pay expenses and expressed her concerns to the nurse at her doctor's office about a month before the baby was expected to arrive. "I'm going to put the baby up for adoption, but I don't know how I'm going to pay the hospital, doctor, and attorney fees," she confided.

"What do you mean?" the nurse asked,

then added, "There are other ways."

"What are you talking about?"

"There's private adoption," the nurse explained and offered to assist her.

A couple was found, and Leta agreed not to see the baby after birth. She heard his first cry, however, and she would carry that memory with her the rest of her life.

Her brother's church sent flowers to encourage her, and when the nurse who had helped her came to visit, she noticed them. "The adoptive parents said for me to look and see if you had any flowers," she told Leta, "and if you didn't, they would send you some."

Postpartum depression struck with a vengeance as she recuperated at her brother's home. At one low point, she reached for the phone and called her friend, the nurse. "How is he doing?" She had to know.

"Well," she was assured, "they had this big party for him when he came home." She felt a little better when she returned the phone to its cradle. Maybe she had done the right thing, she reasoned; at least, she had made someone else happy.

Her sister-in-law stayed with her as she waited to catch her flight back home. The vision of that young woman playing with her own infant daughter filled Leta with sadness and loss as her plane lifted from the ground, and she left her baby boy back in California with strangers.

Journals she kept always noted the same date every year. Today is my son's birthday she would record and mention his age. Perhaps another son would somehow fill that void, she thought, but she had four daughters.

Except for telling her husband, she carried her secret son around inside her heart for several years. She became involved with a pregnant teen through an outreach ministry program in her church. In an effort to connect with the girl, she confided that she understood what she was going through. The unstable teenager, in turn, told Leta's secret to three of her young daughters. To their mother's surprise, they accepted the information without censor.

It had always been a vague thought, but as the years passed, she began to pray that God would help her see her son. She didn't know how to make that happen but continued to pray. She had no idea that when he turned eighteen, he signed a letter of agreement and placed it with the social services in the hope of finding her.

Years passed, and as his half sisters grew into adults, they wanted to know their older brother. They eventually contacted social services in the county where he had been born, and Leta completed the necessary paperwork to show she agreed to being reunited with him.

Within days she received a phone call at work from her husband. A letter had come from social services, he told her; did she want him to open and read it to her? "We have received a consent for contact from you and from your son, Ryan," it said. Ryan's consent letter had been waiting there for six years.

They talked that night for the first time on the phone, and over the next month had long talks as she tried to fill him in on his birth history and tell him how she had always loved him.

One night she arrived home from work around eleven o'clock and was mildly surprised to see each of her daughter's cars there. Judi, her oldest, met her in the front yard and handed her the portable phone. "Ryan's on the phone," she said.

"Hey, whatcha doin'?" she began and they

chatted as she entered the house and then proceeded to her bedroom, where another daughter silently beckoned. She pushed the door open and gasped as she saw her son sitting on her bed, talking to her on the phone. She grabbed him and hugged him as the tears streamed down her face.

Ryan had sent pictures of himself and was readily recognizable. He was surprised, however, when one of his half sisters picked him up at the airport. All his life, he confided, he had looked around and wondered but never found anyone who resembled him. For the first time, here was someone who looked like him.

Meeting each other hasn't brought the "happily ever after" ending as Leta had hoped. They struggled with getting to know each other. She sought and got his forgiveness for giving him away, but he can't bring himself to return her declarations of love.

She finds she has to give him "a good lettin' alone," as she puts it, when weeks go by without hearing from him. He did call her on that first Mother's Day and has visited a few more times. He has met his birth father.

"Lord, was it too early?" she sometimes prays aloud when she gets discouraged and finds comfort in a homespun remark from a friend: "If it wasn't time for you to find him, it was close enough to where it scared it to death," the no-nonsense lady believes.

When Leta looks back over more than twenty-five years to that troubling time in her life, she could dwell on the what-ifs and if-onlys, but she doesn't. What she sees clearly is the hand of God upon a bad situation and is grateful not to have weathered her longtime storm alone.

> *He honors the childless wife in her home;*
> *he makes her happy by giving her children.*
> PSALM 113:9
> GOOD NEWS BIBLE

A BABY OF HER OWN

"You're not praying hard enough." Christie winced inwardly as the thoughtless words stung. How could anyone say such a thing to her? *You're not going through this,* she thought, not for the first time. She felt so abandoned in her storm-tossed world of barrenness. Even

God seemed to have let her down.

For two years she weathered an infertility nightmare of specialists, painful procedures, disappointments, and debt. She and her husband, Rocco, had come to hate life. Their friends were having babies. Other family members were having babies. Even people who abused their children were having babies. She knew because she worked every day as a case manager with these kids. Why was life so unfair? What had they done to deserve this? So many unanswerable questions plagued her thoughts.

This last attempt to have a baby had been the worst. The doctor had offered two choices: artificial insemination or in vitro fertilization (IVF). They chose the latter. Already thousands of dollars in debt, they borrowed $10,000 more and pinned their hopes on the granddaddy of fertility treatments.

In vitro fertilization is a procedure whereby Christie's eggs were commingled with prepared sperm in a sterile laboratory setting. The fertilized eggs were then implanted in her uterus.

Four of the tiny embryos were placed in Christie's womb and, for the first time, she felt like a mother. She gave each of them a name. Two weeks later, however, a phone call informed her that none of the four embryos had implanted. She wasn't pregnant. Her four babies, her only babies ever, were dead.

She looked at the petri dish the clinic had given her, the one where her eggs had been fertilized. Someone had stuck a smiley face in the bottom. She couldn't look at it anymore. To her, it now represented a coffin. How dare they tell her they were just eggs? They had been her babies, and she felt like she was losing her sanity, too.

For two more years their life seemed to be stuck on an emotional roller coaster. Every month she hoped that would be the one when she learned she was finally pregnant. It was always the same, trying to convince herself it was going to happen, urging Rocco to keep the faith. Every day she smiled at him, then cried by herself so he wouldn't know how she grieved for her unborn children. She didn't know he was doing the same thing.

Then they were offered a new procedure, one with a money-back guarantee. She let herself hope once again. During the preprocedure examination, however, the doctor discovered what he referred to as a mass. After a frightening round of appointments: ultrasound, CAT scan, and shuffling from one doctor to another, she was sent to a specialist two hours away.

The sign said Cancer Institute when they located the building containing his office. Cancer? No one had mentioned cancer to her. They didn't know, the doctor informed her, but if the mass on her ovary proved malignant when they operated, they would have to do a total hysterectomy.

Still groggy from the anesthesia, she awoke to find Rocco at her side. Her first question confirmed her worst fear. They had done the full hysterectomy. Now she faced a series of chemotherapy treatments. Precautionary, the doctor said, to be sure the cancer was completely removed.

They told her to take three months off from work, but she returned three weeks after the surgery because she felt she would go mad with too much time alone to think.

"You don't need a baby," the children she worked with told her, "we're your kids." Their awkward attempts to comfort her touched her heart.

She hated taking a shower because there would always be wads of her long blond hair stuck to the drain. Every morning started the same way: Wake, take a shower, cry, and go to work. Some days she didn't care if they had gotten all the cancer or not because she might as well be dead.

The hysterectomy had brought closure, however, to the depressing attempts and failures to conceive. As she began to feel better physically, she made a conscious decision not to let what the cancer had done to her life take control. She would find a way out of the dark clouds that had hung over their life for the past five years and, with God's help, she would somehow be a mother.

They started proceedings for a private adoption. Her spirit soared as she prepared a nursery and made plans. A week before the baby was due to be born, however, the girl changed her mind and left the state. Again, the crushing disappointment threatened to claim her soul.

Friends who were involved in foster care with the hope of adoption suggested they try that route to parenthood. This sounded risky. What if another birth mother decided she wanted her child back? What if they raised a child only to lose him or her to biological parents? After much thought and prayer, they decided to take one more step in blind faith and try. She knew they could be good parents if they were just given a chance.

The representative for the county agency on foster care told them they had a child, a two-month-old boy, with little chance the parents would be involved. The first time they saw Dominic, the agency room was filled with case-workers, the foster parents who were caring for him, Rocco's mother, and the adoption consultant. Christie barely noticed the crowd, however, because her eyes were on the blue-eyed, fair-haired baby who looked a lot like her.

She tried not to love him in case something went wrong again, but as she held his soft, cuddly body in her arms, she couldn't help the telltale tears that betrayed just how much she really cared. *This must be what a biological mother feels the first time she holds her child*, she thought. The hour sped by much too fast, and it was hard to return him to the foster parents. She wanted to grab him back and take him home.

The foster mother brought Dominic on the day Christie and Rocco finally got to become parents. "Hold out your arms," she instructed, and when Christie lovingly reached out and received her new son, the kind woman said, "Happy Mother's Day."

They discovered Dominic had a five-year-old half sister in foster care. After prayerful consideration, they decided to bring Kessla into their family, too. They began with ever-lengthening visits to get to know the sad little girl who had already experienced too many storms of her own.

With Christie's training in helping children of abuse, she feels she can make a difference in the child's life. It will mean giving up her career for awhile, but she believes it is worth it to be a full-time mother.

They found that God not only blessed the life they had come to hate, but in the midst of the storm, He blessed them abundantly. And two unwanted children will have the chance at a better life.

> *My father and mother may abandon me, but the LORD will take care of me.*
>
> PSALM 27:10
> GOOD NEWS BIBLE

CHILDHOOD LOST

Joni's early childhood memories are of loving parents and happy times, an unlikely setting for a devastating life-changing storm. She was born when her mother was thirty-nine and her three siblings were grown or nearly grown, thus she spent a lot of time alone with her parents.

Her father held a high position with the *Birmingham News,* and she describes her family as upper middle class, her material advantages making her the envy of her friends. She remembers her parents as being happy with each other. The three of them went to church together every Sunday, where the devout little girl gave her life to God.

There had been a frightening incident when Joni was a small child in kindergarten. She came home from school one day to find police cars, fire trucks, and paramedics at her house. Her father met her in the front yard and picked her up in his arms. He told her something terrible had happened and took her inside to her mother's bedroom.

Her mother lay in the bed, badly bruised and unable to sit up. They had been robbed that day, she learned. When the maid heard her mother screaming, she found her in the basement, chained and hanging from a beam. She had been about to choke to death. This wasn't the first act of violence that had touched them. Before Joni could remember, there had been another robbery, that time with a gun held to their heads.

They built their dream house and moved away from the house with all the bad memories. When Joni was ten, however, little things started happening to them again. It began as nuisance things like sugar in the gas tank, but quickly escalated to more threatening proportions. They were robbed again. The police came, and the story was in the newspapers. Her father bought a gun.

Then one night Joni awoke to her father screaming, "I'm gonna kill 'em. I'm gonna kill 'em!" As she slid out of her bed, she noticed wet footprints on her carpet as though someone had walked through dewy grass before entering her room.

Her father was in the hallway still screaming as she ran out. He kept trying to aim the gun while her mother attempted to calm him. He couldn't see, and he looked as though something had splattered all over him.

Whoever had broken into the house and left the footprints in Joni's room had thrown acid on her father. He spent the next five months traveling back and forth to the eye foundation, and Joni missed a lot of school.

He eventually recovered from his burns, but shortly after that he became ill. Doctors couldn't find anything wrong with him to explain the nausea, pain, and vomiting. He became so ill they had to admit him to the hospital where tests eventually revealed arsenic poisoning.

When Joni thinks of her childhood from that point on, it is overshadowed with scandal and gossip. Everyone talked about them.

One morning her mother told her she was going to visit her father at the hospital and took Joni to stay with her aunt. Later that afternoon the house started filling up until Joni counted at least forty people there. Whenever they looked at her they started crying. "What is wrong? Why are you crying?" the frightened child kept asking, but no one would say.

Her aunt took her back to the bedroom. "Something terrible has happened to your mama, and she won't be with us anymore," she said. *A car wreck on the way to the hospital,* Joni thought, and they let her believe that.

Finally Joni's sister came. "Where is she? Where is she?" Joni could hear her asking before she saw her. It was from her sister that Joni learned that the cause of her father's illness was poison and that their mother was the prime suspect for attempting his murder.

Her mother had left a note that said she was tortured to the point that she could go on no longer and that she would never do anything to hurt her husband. Then she put a hose on the exhaust of her car and took her own life.

Joni had to go with her two sisters and brother to tell her father what had happened. "You've got to be a big girl and not cry," they warned her.

"I can't go in there," she sobbed, so they went in without her.

They returned a few minutes later and said her father wanted her. His body was partially paralyzed, and he could barely talk. He could manage to write feebly, and he scribbled that he wanted her on the bed with him. They lifted her up and placed his arms around her. He whispered, "Don't worry, it's going to be okay. When I get out of this hospital we'll get us a place together. Now don't you worry because we're going to be just fine." She believed him, but a month later he died.

Her parents had been her whole life. She never even wanted to stay overnight with a friend because she would rather be with them. Now they were both gone, and she didn't even have a chance to tell either one good-bye or to see her home again. Joni went to live with her oldest sister, Jane, and her two children.

Her whole life had changed so abruptly, and she felt angry. "I lost my way," she says of that time. "I didn't know who I was anymore." She hated everyone, especially her mother for leaving her when she had a choice. And she hated God. How could He do this to a little girl who trusted Him? the child demanded of heaven.

Resentment simmered inside her and gradually spilled over as rebellion when she became an adolescent. She started skipping school and hanging out with the wrong crowd. They introduced her to cigarettes and then alcohol. Although her sister was kind to her, she attempted to run away from home.

Maybe a father figure would help, her older

sister decided, and sent her to live with her other sister and brother-in-law in Montgomery. At first it went well. Then one night while playing a game that involved hiding under a blanket, her brother-in-law behaved inappropriately.

Although she was never raped, for over a year she lived in fear of his advances. She locked her door at night to stop him from coming into her room. She didn't know what to do and didn't think anyone would believe her if she told what he was doing to her. A secret part of her mind thought she deserved to be treated badly. Her mother had left her, she reasoned, and now this man was terrorizing her. There must be something wrong with her.

When she was sixteen she was sent for counseling, but it proved disastrous. The psychologist wanted Joni to open up to her, but Joni simply stared stubbornly at the woman. The woman stared back, and hours passed in complete silence as the two glared at each other. She would never amount to anything, the psychologist told Joni's sister, and advised her to just write her off.

She acted out her anger and frustration the only way she knew how by behaving badly again. This time she added drugs to her bad girl image. She graduated from high school and eventually college as well, but still the anger raged inside her.

For a long time she felt no sense of wrong about what she was doing. Slowly, however, a still, small voice began to pierce the havoc inside her. *You don't need to be here,* the voice would say, or *This is wrong. You need to get your life together.*

She married and after nine years finally became pregnant. She sees that as the time her life began to turn around. "God began to place people in my life," she says. One of these was a neighbor who invited her to church. Vineyard, a nondenominational church, provided the background for her to renew her relationship with God. Almost immediately, the feelings she had known as a happy child came back to her.

"I thought God had left me," she confides, "but I heard His voice saying to me, 'I never left you. I was always with you. I will never leave you. I'm your father. I'm your mother. I'm your sister. I'm everything you need.'"

Joni's oldest sister, Jane, came the closest to being her surrogate mother. She worked as an office administrator at the hospital where Joni was scheduled to deliver her baby in April.

In February, Jane fell and suffered a badly broken leg. Joni teased her that she would have to come to her baby tea on crutches. Then suddenly she was gone, a victim of a blood clot. Joni was devastated and the old dark feelings threatened to engulf her again. This time, however, there was a new life growing inside her. She knew she had to go on. "He knew I couldn't survive losing another person in my life like that without giving me new life," Joni says. She believes that is why it took so long for her to get pregnant, that it was God's timing.

She worried how it would be when the baby was born. Would it be sad because Jane wouldn't be there? Would she be swept up in postpartum depression? "It turned out to be the most unbelievable day of my life," she remembers.

Her other sister and brother came to the hospital as well as nephews, nieces, and several cousins. Jane had been greatly admired at the hospital, and now they let special circumstances prevail and allowed the whole family to come.

The doctor who delivered Joni's baby girl was a Christian. As soon as the birth was over, he offered a special prayer right there in the delivery room for the new baby and new mother and for Jane and the family and friends who missed her so much. "Everyone cried," Joni says. "This baby brought the whole family together. We had all been through so much misery, death, and tragedy; and now we had this new life. It was God healing us."

"Since then," she adds, "everything in my life has just fallen into place." She felt God pushing her to teach. She thought He meant Sunday school, but it just didn't work out. Then a job teaching three-year-old kindergartners in a Christian school seemed to simply fall into her lap. "He's healing me so much every day with this school and these people," she confides.

She is able to look back over her storm-tossed life and recognize the blessings that have been wrought from a bad time. She has forged a deeper compassion and sympathy for others and feels she would someday like to work with children who are having problems.

To see this pretty lady with the bright smile today, one would never suspect the tragedy of her background. Friends often ask her how she survived. "Through God," she tells them, "and I'm still making it."

LIFE-CHANGING STORMS PRAYER

Father God, it's storming again,
not just a shower of pesky problems,
but a gully washer that swept away hope and
undermined our faith. Trouble has twisted life
into knots, and it takes more than a good night's
sleep to erase the tiredness from our faces.
Only You can help this time.
We cling so desperately to our storm-battered
trust. Please penetrate the storm that holds
us in its grasp, Lord, and set us on higher
ground where we may be able to put the
pieces of our life back together again.
Touch the madness that claims our days
and rework this cataclysmic disturbance
into something for Your good.
In Your Son's name we pray.
Amen.

I walked a mile with Pleasure.
She chattered all the way,
But left me none the wiser
For all she had to say.

I walked a mile with Sorrow,
And ne'er a word said she;
But, oh, the things I learned from her
When Sorrow walked with me!

ROBERT BROWNING HAMILTON

LOOK FOR THE RAINBOW

Rainbows happen when sunlight penetrates the storm clouds. It takes raindrops to place a rainbow in the sky, and oftentimes it takes teardrops to make a smile deeper and brighter.

Storms are never gentle, and it is the nature of life to not run smoothly for long. If not for the storms, however, we would never know the special beauty found in a rainbow.

Where is our faith in the storm? When we behold it, even a brief glimpse of God in our own personal turmoil, it is better than any pot of gold one could ever find at the end of that colorful arch. The rainbow and the hope it symbolizes are more than enough through any storm.

> *I am putting my bow in the clouds. It will be the sign of my covenant with the world. Whenever I cover the sky with clouds and the rainbow appears, I will remember my promise to you and to all the animals that a flood will never again destroy all living beings.*
>
> GENESIS 9:13–15
> GOOD NEWS BIBLE

> *He who has ears, let him hear.*
>
> MATTHEW 11:15 NIV

SILENT STORM

It must have felt to Winora's parents like one of life's storms had become stuck in a perpetual rainy season when their baby girl was born deaf.

Never having heard even the sound of her

own first breath, this child of silence grew up not missing that which she didn't have. She married and raised ten children. She even joined in their music, beating out time through the vi brations she could feel.

By the time she was a great-grandmother, science and technology had made great contributions to medicine, and her grandchildren decided to have her fit with a hearing aid. Maybe it would help her and maybe it wouldn't, but they insisted she try.

Several of her family members gathered in her home to see what would happen when the man fitted her with the tiny apparatus. One descendent, however, was too small to appreciate the impact of the moment, and her little great-granddaughter began to fuss.

As her mother attempted unsuccessfully to still the crying infant, the hearing aid man inserted the device into Winora's ears and made adjustments.

"What is that?!" the old woman indicated.

The first sound this mother of ten and grandmother of many more ever heard was her great-granddaughter's cry. She wept for joy.

SNOW ON SNOW

Snow on snow,
the sky's largess
makes the road
a slippery mess.

Snow on snow,
the drifts grow deep,
canceled plans,
promises keep.

Snow on snow,
with sleet and rain,
shovel and scrape
to deep back pain.

Snow on snow,
lawn's far below it.
As long as it snows
I don't have to mow it.

DIAMOND DUST

Last night
a diamond came flying by.

I know. I know. I know.
There are tiny bits of diamond dust
all over the snow.

CORINNE CRONLUND

THE INVITATION

The pleasure of your company,
The wind seems to call,
As wondering eyes watch
The first snowfall.

Swirling, inviting,
Yet awesomely still,
Each flake seems to beckon
As it piles on her sill.

Bittersweet longing
Stirs in her soul,
To answer the call
Of this wonderland dole.

A winter storm's bounty
Is there for the claim

With sleigh rides, and ski slides
And a fox-n-geese game.

Snowmen to fashion
Are awaiting her touch,
But, no. . .
Thank you very much.

Fluffy white snowfalls
Are for remembering when
For a little girl locked
In an old woman's skin.

*The Lord is my rock, my fortress, and my
deliverer, my God, my rock in whom I
take refuge, my shield, and the horn of
my salvation, my stronghold. I call upon
the Lord, who is worthy to be praised. . . .*
PSALM 18:2–3 NRSV

AFRAID OF THUNDERSTORMS

(Thanks to my friend, Mary Herron,
for sharing her story with me.)

A clap of thunder awakened Mary to her worst nightmare. She quickly pulled the blankets over her head and covered her ears with the pillow, but it was no use. Though she couldn't see the lightning, she knew it was there flickering into her room like a serpent's tongue. And, even though slightly muted, she could still hear the jarring crash of thunder that vibrated in the pit of her stomach as though making fun of her pounding heart.

The angels are bowling, she told herself over and over, but that old explanation she remembered when being held firmly on her mother's lap as a child didn't work anymore. There was no safe lap when you were a teenager and still terrified of thunderstorms.

Her fear seemed silly when she awoke again in the morning to sunlight beaming through the same window that had allowed the lightning to invade her room just hours before. Would her friends laugh at her if they knew her secret fear?

Her irrational fear came to mind that next Sunday when she listened to the minister's sermon. "God can do anything if we have faith and believe," he had insisted. Did that include overcoming her terror of thunder and lightning? she wondered. Did she dare ask Him to take away that fear?

All week those questions kept nagging her thoughts. The next Sunday the pastor inquired of his flock, "Did you ask God to take a concern from your heart?" Although it was addressed to the whole congregation, she felt the words were meant just for her.

That afternoon she took a walk along the beach that bordered the Maine town where she lived. She needed to pin down the scattered fragments of her thoughts and secure them with some answers. Could God possibly bother with the simple problems of a young girl?

Waves rolled and splashed against rocks while gulls clamored overhead producing comfortable sounds that felt like music to her troubled thoughts. She found a rock and sat upon it to ponder her problem further. Would God, the Creator of this immense sea she now gazed upon, bother with such a silly fear? Again she wondered, did she dare ask

Him to take it away?

A burst of salty spray against her rocky seat told her the tide was coming in, and it was time to leave. Before she left this place she knew she had to take, for her, a giant leap of faith. "Lord," she said aloud, tilting her head skyward while her long auburn hair tangled in the wind, "please take my fear of thunderstorms away."

She held tightly to the minister's words as she twisted the radio dial each morning, searching for a weather report. Ask and believe, he had said. That was all that stood between her and her phobia.

One morning her mother inquired, "Didn't you wake up last night during the storm? It shook the whole house with its clashing." She could feel a warm sense of joy rise from deep within her. Could it be? Had her prayer really been answered?

That weekend, as she walked to her part-time job, she noticed dark clouds forming on the horizon. She walked faster, but the wind that moved the storm clouds was quicker. Rain pelted her face and arms, and a zigzag arrow of lightning shot across the sky just ahead of the thunder.

She hurried to shelter to escape a drenching, but her heart wasn't pounding. No knots formed in her stomach. She stood in amazement and watched as the thunderstorm continued, but those old feelings of fear were gone. A brief prayer rose automatically to her lips, and she whispered, "Thank You, God."

But all who find safety in you will rejoice; they can always sing for joy. Protect those who love you; because of you they are truly happy.

PSALM 5:11
GOOD NEWS BIBLE

THE BLOCK OF WOOD

A small block of wood sits on my desk, and I treasure it. It measures about three inches high and two inches wide. Much of the inside has been made into a hollowed-out circle. It holds pens, paper clips, and any other small object that happens to need a place to save it from becoming clutter.

I bought it not because I need one more

thing to take up space on my desk, but because of what it says. Writer's Block, someone has carefully written on its side with a wood-burning tool. Besides enjoying the pun, I prize this little piece of wood because of where it has been.

My pen holder was cut, carefully sanded smooth (making it a pleasure to rub one's fingers over its side), and lettered inside a prison workshop. Its maker was incarcerated in a state prison. I bought it, while vacationing in Maine, from a special store that is operated by the prisoners. This store is filled with their wooden handiwork, and part of the profit goes to them.

I don't know what crime the man committed who fashioned my little writer's block. Obviously, his was a life of violent storms, or he wouldn't be locked away from society. I like to look at this small block of wood and picture him lovingly working it into something useful. I love it for where it originates, for it reminds me of how even the worst of storms can produce a rainbow in an otherwise ugly sky.

'Tis ever this, when in life's storm
Hope's star to man grows dim,
An angel kneels, in woman's form,
And breathes a prayer for him.

GEORGE POPE MORRIS

STORM BLESSINGS

Count one thousand,
One thousand-one, one thousand-two,
One thousand-three, one thousand-four. . .
My sister and I
Measure the distance of a storm.
Safe on the front porch,
We conquer our fear
As we cuddle close to Mom.

Years and miles away,
In the wake of rare desert rain,
I dance with my husband
On wet Arizona sand,
While the rumble of distant thunder
Keeps time with our footsteps
And cool raindrops
Splash against our skin.

In a few days
Tiny wild flowers
Blossom
From the barren desert sand.

FLORANCE HUSTEDT

The desert will rejoice, and flowers will bloom in the wastelands. The desert will sing and shout for joy; it will be as beautiful as the Lebanon Mountains and as fertile as the fields of Carmel and Sharon. Everyone will see the Lord's splendor, see his greatness and power. Give strength to hands that are tired and to knees that tremble with weakness. Tell everyone who is discouraged, "Be strong and don't be afraid! God is coming to your rescue, coming to punish your enemies."

ISAIAH 35:1–4
GOOD NEWS BIBLE

Let the heavens be glad, and let the earth rejoice. . .Let the sea roar, and all

that fills it; let the field exult, and
everything in it. Then shall the trees of
the forest sing for joy before the LORD,
for he comes. . . .

1 CHRONICLES 16:31–33 NRSV

LET THE EARTH REJOICE

Several people gathered at the cemetery just outside of town in anticipation of the Easter sunrise service. The old graveyard had grown with the town over the decades and spanned an area far up a steep hill. Early morning chill made little puffs of vapor as friends greeted each other and stamped their feet to keep warm.

"Let's climb to the top," someone suggested, either out of a spirit of adventure or the need to keep moving for warmth. His idea caught on, however, and the group made the trek to the top. It proved well worth the effort. That height offered a view of the opposite hill uninterrupted by the tall maple trees that dominated the older part of the cemetery below.

As their singing and prayers penetrated the stillness of the morning, the sun appeared as if on cue. It cast its first beams on the top of the opposing hill, then slid slowly down until it could touch the tops of the maples directly below.

"Look!" Someone pointed, and all eyes rested on one of the old trees. The sun's rays had crept about halfway down the trunk and illuminated a large white cross nestled in the bare limbs. *How did it get there?* everyone wondered, for it was several feet in length and a long way up the tree. And who could have placed it in such a strategic spot for them to view at the perfect moment? Services were traditionally held down there under the old trees. The decision to climb the hill had been made on a whim.

Closer inspection, as they made their way back down the hill, revealed the cross was not man-made. Strong wind and heavy ice or snow from a storm must have broken the large, dead limb in two, which presumably snagged in the surrounding branches as it fell crosswise. Perhaps winter birds had pecked away the outer bark, exposing the white center just far enough on each of the pieces to make a perfect white cross.

It was an awestruck crowd that left the

cemetery that morning. The experience gave new meaning to the words "God's handiwork." A Creator who could not only calm the storms but would also use one to create a work of art in just the right place at just the right time humbled them. "He is risen," they had sung just moments before, "let the earth rejoice." And it had.

> *So all your loyal people should pray to you in times of need; when a great flood of trouble comes rushing in, it will not reach them.*
>
> PSALM 32:6
> GOOD NEWS BIBLE

WHEN YOU WALK THROUGH A STORM

Oscar Hammerstein II wrote a beautiful inspirational song for the 1945 Broadway musical *Carousel* titled "You'll Never Walk Alone." Written while the world was still reeling from WWII, the sentiments in the song's message touched a lot of anxious hearts not only in the United States but Great Britain, as well.

The song advises us to walk on through wind and rain even though our dreams are tossed and blown. These are noble and hope-filled words, and while I like the tune a lot, I don't agree with one line: "When you walk through a storm hold your head up high."

A storm isn't a time to hold your head up high unless you want rain in your face. Instead, it is best to bow your head into the wind and rain. The same holds true for all other life storms as well. Bowing your head works better every time.

Dear Lord, sometimes we try prayer
as a last resort when it should be our first.
Thank You for Your wonderful grace
that allows us to mismanage things
our way and then You not only forgive us,
but love us in spite of our failings.
Amen.

It hain't no use to grumble and complain,
It's jest as easy to rejoice;
When God sorts out the weather and
sends rain,
Why rain's my choice.

JAMES WHITCOMB RILEY

SETBACKS

Just when you think you're gaining,
like after a storm,
when it's no longer raining,
A gust of wind
blows water from the trees
and showers you again
from a cloud of leaves.

THE PROMISE

There's a promise of rain in the air.
See the storm clouds the wind has swept?
There's a thirsty garden somewhere
Hoping that promise is kept.

Spring's around the Corner

Spring's around the corner,
The calendar's calling,
But the weatherman says
The barometer's falling.

The Fahrenheit's low,
And snowfall's amounting.
March days slip by,
But who's counting?

*Ask the Lord for rain in the spring of the
year. It is the Lord who sends rain clouds
and showers, making the fields green for
everyone.*

ZECHARIAH 10:1
GOOD NEWS BIBLE

Piñatas

Dark billows of clouds scud across the horizon. Their puffy underbellies resemble great gray piñatas hung from the heavens. Sharp streaks of lightning punch their sides with thunderous abandon until they release their bounty and fat drops of life-giving water spill over the thirsty earth beneath.

Green blades begin to poke through last year's dead grass. Tight-fisted buds unclench, and dried seeds burst into life. The giver of life once again showers His gifts upon a needy world.

> *"Rejoice in the Lord your God! For the rains he sends are tokens of forgiveness. Once more the autumn rains will come, as well as those of spring."*
>
> JOEL 2:23 TLB

> *There by the Ahava Canal I gave orders for us all to fast and humble ourselves before our God and to ask him to lead us on our journey and protect us and our children and all our possessions. I would have been ashamed to ask the emperor for a troop of cavalry to guard us from any enemies during our journey, because I had told him that our God blesses everyone who trusts him, but that he is displeased with and punishes anyone*

*who turns away from him. So we fasted
and prayed for God to protect us, and he
answered our prayers.*

EZRA 8:21–23
GOOD NEWS BIBLE

THE FAST

Tonya worried when her mother announced
she was going to have knee replacement surgery. The older woman was diabetic and required two insulin shots daily, and Tonya knew
how hard it could be for a diabetic to heal. She
had seen a couple of extreme cases where the
patients had ended up losing limbs because of
complications from diabetes after surgery.

Her brother and sister shared her concern,
but their mother remained convinced this was
the best thing to do. The siblings began making
plans to take turns caring for their father, who
was in the early stages of Alzheimer's disease.
Surgery was scheduled for the first Monday in
April, which was about five weeks away.

Church had always been a part of Tonya's
life. Her family attended regularly, and she
sang in choir. It was in choir one Sunday that
she first glimpsed something beyond just

hearing Scripture and trying to live the best life she could. She led the choir that day with her strong sweet voice, and they sang "Jesus, How I Love to Call on Your Name." As she sang, the song became her personal communion with God. "I felt something," she says of that moment. "It was personal."

While in college, she started attending other churches and discovered different forms of praise and worship. She began to tithe.

She couldn't explain the dark clouds of fear she felt for her mother, but the feeling that surgery would be a mistake persisted. "I had heard of people fasting and praying, but I had never done it," she admits. She didn't know where else to turn, however, so she began this ancient act of humbling oneself before God.

She combined prayer and partial fasting, eating only between the hours of three and seven in the afternoon, and limiting the selection and amounts. She drank plenty of water. "When I got hungry," she confides, "I would just sing a joyful song."

Fasting, it is believed, cleanses one of sin and allows a sharper sensitivity to spiritual things. The Bible tells of this approach to seeking God's presence by many persons, including Jesus.

On the Friday before the scheduled surgery, Tonya's cousin, who is a nurse, called her. "Why are you letting your mother go through with this surgery?" he asked. "Do you know the chances of her bouncing back from this and how extensive the rehab is going to be?"

She assured him she knew but that her mother was insistent. She also told him about her fasting and prayers. "It's not too late," she said. "The surgery is not scheduled until Monday."

After she hung up the phone, she went for a walk. "It's not too late," she repeated her words in a prayer. "It's in Your hands."

A short while later, while talking to a friend on the phone, her call waiting beeped. It was her mother's doctor's office. They had been unable to reach her mother, the nurse told her, but the routine pre-op EKG had shown an abnormality. Until this could be further checked with a cardiologist, the surgery would have to be postponed.

"When she told me that," Tonya confides, "I knew it was nothing but the Lord stopping this surgery. He put this little glitch in there to show up. There's nothing wrong with my mother's heart."

She is convinced her fasting was not in vain, and it appears she might be right. A stress test revealed no problem with her mother's heart. She doesn't mention the knee problems anymore, either. There are a lot of ways to weather a storm. For Tonya, it is going beyond a craving for food and satisfying an inner hunger for God. When fortified in that way, she feels confident to meet whatever storm life may bring.

HOPE

Have you ever
told your dream
to the first evening star
as you shivered in the chill of the night,
confident your wish was heard?

Have you ever
tossed a coin into a fountain,
trusting in a fate
you could buy for a penny?

Have you ever
chased a rainbow
and been lost in the midst

with a soggy feeling inside,
but you kept on looking
for the pot of gold?

Have you ever
emptied your heart
before God
and found it full of doubt,
yet your soul stood on tiptoe
to knock again
at heaven's door?

Have you ever
bound your heart's desire
with a fine thread of hope
and waited?

Have you?
Ever?

And it is he who will supply all your
needs from his riches in glory, because of
what Christ Jesus has done for us.
PHILIPPIANS 4:19 TLB

Lauren has suffered with a serious heart problem since birth. Besides the special care she needed, her parents struggled to pay for her medications, which cost over $400 a month.

One thing a child who has to limit her activity can do is look at books, and a family friend showered the little girl with volumes of them ever since she was born. Many of these her mother, Meloney, set aside until the youngster could grow into them. Such was the case with the Precious Moments Bible, given to her while she was still a baby.

A toddler's Bible, a preschool Bible, and even a Children of Color Bible showed signs of wear as the little girl grew, while the Precious Moments Bible remained untouched. Her mother felt it was just too advanced for her yet.

The spring when Lauren was four, the apartment complex where they lived caught on fire. Though the blaze started three apartments down from theirs, it spread fast. Fortunately, no one was hurt, but most of their home was in ruins. Flames completely destroyed their kitchen, while the living room and master bedroom suffered extensive water damage. Lauren's room along with all her belongings, however, remained oddly untouched.

They lost a lot in the fire, and by July the financial strain had become too much. Lauren's hospital and doctor bills plus the regular rent, household bills, and credit card payments far exceeded their budget. Although Meloney's husband worked two jobs, his hours had been cut back. There was just no money to pay for the eleven different medications Lauren took every month. All they could do was pray about it.

Meloney usually had the prescriptions refilled before the fifth of each month, but by the eleventh there was no medicine left and no money to buy more. Feeling helpless to change the situation, she decided to take Lauren to the small park down the hill from their home where they might escape the dark cloud of worry for a little while.

Lauren became engrossed in watching a child play with a new puppy while the mother chatted with Meloney. Although the conversation was casual, Meloney had a hard time concentrating on what the woman said.

Precious! Precious! The odd word kept interrupting her thoughts over and over again. It was just one word, but it wouldn't stop jamming the circuits of her mind. *I don't know anybody by the name of Precious,* she reasoned with the silent voice clamoring inside her head.

As soon as they returned home from the park, Lauren asked if she could have one of her books. They were kept high on a long shelf at the back of her closet, and as she reached for one, Meloney asked, "This one?"

"No."

"This one?" she asked again as her fingers slid to the next.

"No."

Finally Lauren decided on her selection, and her mother carefully pulled it from the row. As she did, another book several spaces down the shelf tumbled to the floor. The fact that the book had fallen at all surprised her, because it was securely wedged in its place in the long row. She hadn't touched it or any of the books near it.

When she bent down to pick it up, she discovered the shrink-wrap that bound it had broken on impact, allowing the pages to separate. Tucked between the leaves where it lay opened was a small stack of money. Astonished at what had just happened, she was dumbfounded further when she read the title: Precious Moments

Bible. "Precious" was the word she had received in the park minutes before.

How could a shrink-wrapped book contain money between its pages? Wasn't that all done by machines in a factory somewhere? Where had it come from? Who put it there? Could it have anything to do with why Lauren's room had been mysteriously spared in the fire? When she turned to her grandfather for answers he said, "God works in mysterious ways and has His own way of doing things. Everything that happens, happens for a reason, and God is in control of that. He knew that one day you wouldn't have the money for that baby's medicine."

"As far as I am concerned," says Meloney, "it was a miracle." The amount of money in the book totaled $450, just what they needed to pay for Lauren's prescriptions.

LOOK FOR THE RAINBOW PRAYER

Lord of life and giver of abundant life,
we are overwhelmed by Your goodness
and mercy. Forgive us, please,
for the dark corners of doubt, worry,
and fear that creep into our being.
Thank You for those rainbow glimpses of hope
and encouragement that keep us going.
There will always be storms, Father. Help us
to weatherproof our faith so that we may
hold firm and look for You in all things.
Amen.

So now, since we have been made right
in God's sight by faith in his promises,
we can have real peace with him because
of what Jesus Christ our Lord has done
for us. For because of our faith, he has
brought us into this place of highest
privilege where we now stand, and we
confidently and joyfully look forward to
actually becoming all that God has had
in mind for us to be.

ROMANS 5:1–2 TLB

Inspirational Library

Beautiful purse/pocket-size editions of Christian classics bound in flexible leatherette. These books make thoughtful gifts for everyone on your list, including yourself!

When I'm on My Knees   The highly popular collection of devotional thoughts on prayer, especially for women.
Flexible Leatherette. $4.97

The Bible Promise Book   Over 1,000 promises from God's Word arranged by topic. What does God promise about matters like: Anger, Illness, Jealousy, Love, Money, Old Age, and Mercy? Find out in this book!
Flexible Leatherette. $3.97

Daily Wisdom for Women   A daily devotional for women seeking biblical wisdom to apply to their lives. Scripture taken from the New American Standard Version of the Bible.
Flexible Leatherette. $4.97

My Daily Prayer Journal   Each page is dated and features a Scripture verse and ample room for you to record your thoughts, prayers, and praises. One page for each day of the year.
Flexible Leatherette. $4.97

Available wherever books are sold.
Or order from:

Barbour Publishing, Inc.
P.O. Box 719
Uhrichsville, OH 44683
http://www.barbourbooks.com

If you order by mail, add $2.00 to your order for shipping.
Prices are subject to change without notice.